COVID-19 and the Case Against Neoliberalism

Mark Boyle · James Hickson ·
Katalin Ujhelyi Gomez

COVID-19 and the Case Against Neoliberalism

The United Kingdom's Political Pandemic

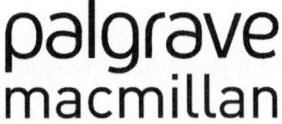

Mark Boyle
Department of Geography
National University of Ireland,
Maynooth
Kildare, Ireland

James Hickson
The Heseltine Institute for Public
Policy, Practice and Place
University of Liverpool
Liverpool, UK

Katalin Ujhelyi Gomez
Institute of Population Health
University of Liverpool
Liverpool, UK

ISBN 978-3-031-18934-0   ISBN 978-3-031-18935-7   (eBook)
https://doi.org/10.1007/978-3-031-18935-7

Cover illustration: © Melisa Hasan

This Palgrave Macmillan imprint is published by the registered company Springer Nature Switzerland AG
The registered company address is: Gewerbestrasse 11, 6330 Cham, Switzerland

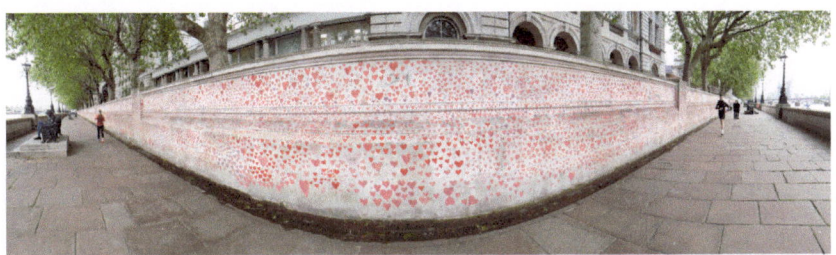

Plate 1 The National Covid Memorial Wall London (*Source* Pear on Willow CC BY-SA 4.0 24 May 2021)

The National Covid Memorial Wall on South Bank of the river Thames in London, UK, was created as a collaboration between the COVID-19 Bereaved Families for Justice and Led By Donkeys groups. Adorning the Wall are over 150,000 red and pink hearts inscribed with personal messages of loss and memorialisation. The Wall was painted by 1500 volunteers starting on 29 March 2021 over a ten-day period. Plans are afoot to ensure that the Wall remains intact as a permanent reminder of the collective trauma the global family has endured these past years. https://nationalcovidmemorialwall.org/

This book is dedicated to those who lost their lives to COVID-19 and because of COVID-19

We owe it to the families of those whose lives were taken to have the courage to search for, own, and strive to remediate the political progenitors of this global pandemic.

"a misconceived theory can kill" (Sen 1999, 209)

PROLOGUE

This book arose from an interdisciplinary research project on *British neoliberalism and COVID-19* conducted at the Heseltine Institute (University of Liverpool) and intended as a contribution to the (now active, May 2022) independent public inquiry into the UK government's handling of the COVID-19 pandemic.

The Heseltine Institute for Public Policy, Practice and Place is a non-partisan, internationally recognised research institute and thought leader, bringing together expertise from across the University and policy communities, to co-create, impact, and influence public policies for tomorrow's cities. The institute has made a significant contribution to Liverpool City Region's COVID-19 response, including and in particular through its flagship policy briefings series (Series 1 Responding to COVID-19, Series 2 Recovery and Renewal). Further details about the Heseltine Institute and its COVID-19 policy briefings can be accessed at: https://www.liverpool.ac.uk/heseltine-institute/.

Readers should note that whilst substantially original, this manuscript incorporates portions of text from other related papers we have published:

Boyle M., Hickson J. and Ujhelyi Gomez K. (2021). *Change! Strengthening the Resilience of British Cities in Preparation for Future Pandemics.* Heseltine Institute for Public Policy, Practice and Place, University of Liverpool.

Boyle M., Hickson J. and Ujhelyi Gomez K. (2021). *Addendum—Conjectures and Refutations: Further Interrogating Potential Determinants of COVID-19's Geographies*. Heseltine Institute for Public Policy, Practice and Place, University of Liverpool.
Boyle M. (2021). *Human Geography: An Essential Introduction*. Wiley.
Hickson J. (2020). *A Political Theory of Precarious Work*. Unpublished PhD thesis, University of York.

The research base woven throughout this book also derives from a number of cognate-funded projects. The authors wish to thank in particular the Liverpool COVID-19 Partnership Strategic Research Fund (Mark Boyle), the Arts & Humanities Research Council (grant number AH/L503848/1) through the White Rose College of the Arts & Humanities (James Hickson) and the National Institute for Health Research (NIHR) Applied Research Collaboration North West Coast (ARC NWC) at the University of Liverpool (Katalin Ujhelyi Gomez).

Finally, the authors thank Rachel Ballard (Head of Science and Society) and Shreenidhi Natarajan (Project Coordinator) both at Palgrave Macmillan for their professional and efficient handling of the manuscript and the helpful suggestions provided by three anonymous reviewers.

Of course, the views expressed in the book are strictly those of the authors and are not necessarily shared by the supporting institutions or funders identified above.

CONTENTS

List of Figures

LIST OF TABLES

CHAPTER 1

In What Sense a Political Pandemic?

Abstract With public inquiry processes now gathering momentum across the globe (not least in the United Kingdom itself), this book seeks to better understand the meaning and implications of the UK's particularly calamitous encounter with the COVID-19 global pandemic. The book is distinctive in that it mobilises an applied political philosophy perspective to pioneer fresh intellectual resources—both analytical and normative—to advance the thesis that the country's weddedness to an exhausted neoliberal politico-institutional-economic model—and not just, say, epidemiological shocks or political incompetence and bad decision-making—lies at the heart of its poor pandemic outcomes. To set the scene for the remainder of the book, the purpose of this chapter is to elaborate this thesis and establish its principal suppositions, conjectures, and ramifications.

Keywords COVID-19 · Neoliberalism · Public inquiry · Applied political philosophy · United Kingdom · Political geography · Neorepublicanism

INTRODUCTION

The United Kingdom (UK) government has long understood the threat posed by emerging and re-emerging communicable diseases. But it has too readily assumed that the country's comparatively superior health, wealth, and institutional capacities would mitigate risk and enable it to escape the worst: it would, instead, be countries in the Global South that would be most exposed to the brunt of any next generation global pandemic. It has come as something of a shock then that events have unfolded otherwise. Notwithstanding the very significant problems of data availability, variability, and quality, there can be no denying that the UK has found itself amongst those nations most incapacitated by the COVID-19 global pandemic.

This book has its origins in our quest to better understand the UK's encounter with COVID-19, what went wrong and what the UK government will need to fix if it is to—using the jargon of the day—'fail forward', 'build back better', 'emerge stronger', and/or 'recover, reimagine and rebuild'. Our pursuit of the causes of the UK's troubles however has led us to contemplate a number of fundamental questions of more existential import. We have arrived at the conclusion that to understand why the UK has been so injured by COVID-19 it is necessary to first understand the limited and ever deteriorating efficacy of the country's underlying politico-economic-institutional model—and in particular the meaning and implications of its forty-year experiment with neoliberalism. For us, the story of the harm which the pandemic has inflicted on the UK is best construed as the story of an emergent embroilment between an exhausted British neoliberal model and an epidemiological shock event—an entanglement which is proving consequential for both.

The purpose of this book is to elaborate this thesis and reason through its analytical and normative suppositions, conjectures, and ramifications—particularly as they bear on scholarship on each of British neoliberalism, the UK's post-pandemic political dispensation, government plans to build back better and strengthen the country's resilience, and UK public health governance, policy, and practice. In this opening chapter, we set out in greater detail the journey that has taken us to our port of embarkation. Introducing the novel *applied political theory* perspective we adopt, we then identify the new conceptual arsenal we believe this book brings to the table. We end by signposting the structure of the chapters to follow.

In What Sense a Political Pandemic?

A wealthy country boasting very high levels of human development and with strong institutions—including a world-renowned public health care system—the UK had been understood to have completed the epidemiological transition. Yet for most of 2020, the UK government struggled to suppress the SARSnCoV-2 2019 virus, and all too often it lost the battle. Spectators watched with incredulity as the world's fifth largest economy recoiled from reported COVID-19 death rates and levels of excess deaths that at times ranked amongst the worst in the world. From early 2021 the story has taken a turn for the better. A bail out has come in the form of medical science. A cornucopian 'miracle'—an effective vaccine developed at 'warp speed'—has pulled the country back from the brink. But further viral mutation, transmission, and death look inevitable, and at this juncture complete eradication appears to be hopelessly aspirational. We are being advised that we will need to 'learn to live with' (hopefully low transmissible/low virulence) 'endemic' COVID-19 for the foreseeable future.

Whatever transpires, the UK's relatively successful vaccine programme cannot and must not erase or obfuscate prior difficulties; history instructs that societies which rely on technological fixes to engineer themselves out of systemic crises rarely fail forward. If the UK is to emerge from the pandemic stronger, it is imperative that the government gets to the bottom of why the country has toiled so badly with COVID-19 and what these difficulties reveal about what must now be fixed if it is to strengthen resilience in preparation for future pandemic events—and indeed other shocks. To 'build back better' we need to better understand which systems, structures, and institutions are crumbling and why this blight is taking hold. Here we would do well to heed Amartya Sen's sage advice that when it comes to people living in precarity and poverty, 'a misconceived theory can kill'. Causality matters because only precise diagnoses will enable accurate prognosis and effective prescription. The UK can only emerge from the pandemic stronger if it fixes what is broken, but it can only fix what is broken if it understands what is actually broken.

In May 2021, Prime Minister Boris Johnson announced that an independent public inquiry into the UK government's handling of COVID-19 would be held, beginning in Spring 2022. In December 2021, Baroness Heather Hallett was appointed as chair of the inquiry. A UK-wide approach (England, Wales, Scotland, and Northern Ireland) is to be adopted. The purpose of the inquiry is to better understand the impact of COVID-19 on public health and beyond, take stock of the efficacy of the government's response (its disaster risk management, processes, planning and decision-making, and its capacity for 'fast policy'), and extract lessons so that the UK government can prepare for future pandemic events. A problem this wicked is unlikely to yield to cheap explanations; if we are to untangle and appraise the complex brew of potential causal variables which have been mooted, a considerable and painstaking job of work lies ahead.

Clearly, virological factors are likely to have played a significant role in determining the trajectory of the pandemic in the UK; for sure any post-mortem will need to better understand the epidemiological determinants of pathogen lethality, mutation and contagiousness, circulation, diffusion, and exposure. Was the UK exposed to particularly potent and transmissible variants of the virus, and if so why? Could London's global centrality and connectivity have bequeathed an especially dense and porous mesh of capillaries through which the virus was able to travel?

But COVID-19 has been as much a political pandemic as it has been an epidemiological event. Hazards research has long taught us that the risk of harm from a hazard event = exposure (to that hazard event) × vulnerability (underpinning institutional-socio-economic-politico capacity and resilience). We must not confine our attention only to the former. Speaking of the devastation wrought by Hurricane Katrina on New Orleans in 2006, the late Neil Smith argued that there is no such thing as a 'natural disaster': "*In every phase and aspect of a disaster—causes, vulnerability, preparedness, results and response, and reconstruction—the contours of disaster and the difference between who lives and who dies is to a greater or lesser extent a social calculus*" (Smith, 2006, no page). We might paraphrase Smith and insist that there is no such thing as a *natural* pandemic event. It is through the social production of vulnerability and political failure that viral outbreaks scale into pandemics, pandemics translate into disasters, and disasters escalate into catastrophes.

If the UK's initial 'lessons learned' report published jointly by the House of Commons Health and Social Care, and Science and Technology Committees (2021) is anything to go by, it is clear the focus of the public inquiry will be upon government policy. And for good reason. In his book, *The COVID-19 Catastrophe: What's Gone Wrong and How to Stop It Happening Again*, editor-in-chief of the leading medical journal The Lancet Richard Horton (2021) argues that the elevated impact of COVID-19 in the UK reflects at root government incompetence. For Horton, COVID-19 stands as the greatest science policy failure in a generation. The UK government did intervene in a consequential way to protect lives and livelihoods. But it failed to act with the necessary speed, stringency, or coordination to adequately limit the spread of the virus. Measures were often too little, too late; reluctant concessions to the spiralling crisis, rather than positive, proactive, and pre-emptive intervention at the earliest opportunity.

Whilst acknowledging that the UK government, by its actions and inactions, did indeed render the country more vulnerable than it needed to be and placed it at unnecessarily elevated risk, we contend that it would be a cardinal error to confine any inquiry only to government misjudgement, inertia, and ineptitude. What might we miss about the political production (and reproduction) of vulnerability if we confine attention only to public policy failures? It is not just the content, probity, and ramifications of discrete decisions made within the government that must be scrutinised. We must also consider the political theories and political projects that, both implicitly and explicitly, inform government decisions, and shape the choice architectures within which these decisions are made.

And so we might refine our formula: risk = exposure × vulnerability where vulnerability = the efficacy of the underlying politico-economic-institutional model × the efficacy of government's responses. The two domains—politics and policy—are functionally related. Countries will be at heightened risk of harm from COVID-19 (and other such crises) when fundamental socio-structural maladies inflate the impact of public policy choices and in turn public policy choices expose and aggravate structural-institutional precarities. A perfect storm will be the inevitable result: countries that find themselves in this position will be most likely to magnify COVID-19's deleterious impacts. Arguably, the UK falls into this category.

This book will advance the thesis that the UK government's decades-long experimentation with neoliberal institutions, ideas, ideals, and policies stands as a significant determinant of its poor COVID-19 outcomes. But chasing the chronicles of the UK's experience of COVID-19 is as much a point of entry for us as it is a point of terminus. There is a bigger story to tell here. We have written this book as a contribution to scholarship on the odyssey of the UK's neoliberal experiment and indeed the Odyssean travails of neoliberalism and neoliberalism redux more broadly. COVID-19 has intercepted neoliberalism at what appears to be a threshold moment in its life course. The product of forty years of neoliberal rule, politico-economic maladies have weakened the country's resilience and rendered it especially vulnerable to emerging and re-emerging infectious diseases. But COVID-19's public health crisis and its concomitant social and economic aftershocks have in turn attenuated these maladies and catalysed a new moment of recalibration and structuration in the UK's neoliberal model. Alongside approaching neoliberalism as one of a number of potential progenitors of heightened risk of harm from COVID-19 then, we approach COVID-19 as itself a potential progenitor of history; a consequential episode in the tumultuous life of a politico-economic model.

WHAT DOES THIS BOOK OFFER THAT IS NEW?

In forging this argument, we find ourselves in good company. Mobilising variously political philosophy, political economy, political ecology, feminist, and biopolitical framings, there is emerging a body of scholarship which is demonstrating the ways in which neoliberal reform and public health/harm from COVID-19 are interlinked. We are beginning to better understand the causal pathways and feedback loops at work and the ways in which the imbrication of one in the other is giving rise to distinctive co-evolutionary trajectories.

According to Standring and Davies (2020) and Navarro (2020), prior neoliberal policies, boom and bust economics, fiscal consolidation and austerity, and the privatisation of health services, have denuded the Italian, Spanish, and US governments' capacity to respond swiftly and effectively to COVID-19. Likewise, in their comparative analysis of early stage responses to the pandemic in the UK, the US, Germany, and South Korea, Mellish et al. (2020) contend that the excessive ideological weddedness of the UK and USA rendered these countries particularly vulnerable. For Giroux (2021) and Sparke and Williams (2022, 16), the pandemic has "at once exposed, exploited and exacerbated" the health damaging legacies of neoliberal rule: "neoliberal plans, policies and practices advanced globally in the name of promoting wealth have proved disastrous in terms of protecting health in the context of the pandemic". Sultana (2021, 447) meanwhile makes a compelling case for considering together—through a feminist lens—the overlapping global crises of neoliberalism, socio-ecological and climate change, and the COVID-19 pandemic, noting therein the ways in which each has "co-created new challenges, vulnerabilities, and burdens, as well as reinforcing old ones". In another contribution Glover and Maani (2020) question the extent to which the UK's COVID-19 response—and its failures—will in time come to be seen as a moment of 'peak neoliberalism'. In a similar vein, Saad-Filho (2020) has interrogated the extent to which COVID-19 has forced governments into such a massive Keynesian stimulus that the pandemic might in fact signal the end of neoliberalism. For Šumonja (2021) and Ryan, however, disaster capitalism and neoliberalism redux are the more likely outcomes.

So what is new about this book?

Ours is the first book length monograph that (to the best of our knowledge) forges this species of argument in the company of *applied political theory* and equipped with this scholarly tradition's analytical and methodological tools. As such, our ambition is to develop a distinctive and novel rendering of the nexus between neoliberalism and country level COVID-19 outcomes and thereby to supplement, augment, and enrich—and not just embellish, fortify, and consolidate—existing literature and build capacity amongst scholars, politicians, and practitioners who believe that the neoliberalism-COVID-19 nexus lies at the heart of the UK's poor pandemic outcomes.

We explain why it is important to interrogate the political theories that underpin public decision-making as well as to understand their secular actually existing groundings and situated and contested structuration. We call attention in particular to the pivotal importance of the concept of 'freedom' and critique the work that neoliberalism's peculiar and parochial concept of freedom does—and indeed prohibits—in the world. We populate this critique with new analytic and normative content by juxtaposing neoliberalism's philosophy of freedom with an alternative neorepublican philosophy of freedom. We revisit this dualism throughout the text, demonstrating at every turn how freedom should not be thought of as antithetical to social democracy but instead as its foundational pillar. We argue that British neoliberalism has (overtly and by stealth) taken custody of the concept freedom and in so doing has hindered the country's capacity to deal with shock events.

We have invested heavily in settling upon a compelling analytical entrée. We believe that if we are to make sense of the UK's deleterious encounter with COVID-19 we must ask first: what exact analytical problem does this encounter present? If we fail to frame and specify the problem adequately we will surely fail to discern and ascribe priority to the progenitors that matter most, will fail to understand these progen-itors in their richness and complexity, and will go looking for solutions and remedies in the wrong places.

So what is our port of embarkation? *We have chosen to think in terms of the tumultuous struggles of fallible leaders who, operating on a canvas produced by forty years of actually existing British neoliberalism (socio-economic-political-cultural legacies) and within the rubric of actually existing British neoliberal policy mentalities (politico-institutional logics) have been called upon to respond to an epic shock event for which there has been no playbook.*

To help us progress this meta-framing, we invoke the central idea of 'choice architectures'—or what Jacques Ranciére (2004) refers to as the 'partition (distribution) of the sensible (permissible'). Political actors, enmeshed in historical and parochial political logics, overwhelmed by an epidemiological disaster without precedent and facing cognitive over-load and disablement, mobilise what intellectual and normative resources they have at their disposal to fashion a 'common sense' response. These resources—applied political theories and the choice architectures they spawn—both enable and constrain what these leaders are able to think and do.

Stated this baldly, this reasoning is not especially illuminating. It becomes more productive however when accompanied by three further analytic moves.

a. *Treating structure, agency, and structuration as co-equals*

We call attention to the ways in which different political philosophies—albeit in highly variegated, contextual, contingent, and contested ways—bequeath different public health sensibilities and permissible pandemic management options. But even as historical actors, it is agenic political leaders who embrace, domesticate, translate, and localise choice architec-tures and who in the final analysis make public policy choices and life and death decisions. And so whilst anchoring political constructs play a central role in creating conditions of possibility for pandemic manage-ment strategies, the enactment of these strategies too plays a central role in the situated structuration of the underpinning political common sense.

Readers will immediately notice that we are thus refusing to give analytical priority to any one of *structure, agency, and structuration*. In fact our narrative arc seeks to hold all three in play at least as insightful categories of analysis.

- <u>Structure</u>. Whilst recognising that they only ever exist in actually existing form and are never truly hegemonic, we insist upon studying the logical integrity and coherent disciplinary technes of political theories and their choice architectures. The power of knowledge is what enables knowledge to become power. If not with reference to their allegiance to a coherent underlying political metaphysics, how else can we explain why so many western OECD governments got it so badly wrong?
- <u>Agency</u>. Whilst we recognise that all political leaders are embedded, situated, and historical actors, we take seriously their agency and autonomy and by implication their accountability. Whilst (deeply) functionally inter-related, there remains a distance to travel between choice architectures and actually existing choices. How else can we explain why not all neoliberal states performed badly and not all poor performers are neoliberal in their ideology?
- <u>Structuration</u>. Whilst treating structure and agency as meaningful categories of analysis, we recognise that ontologically, political theories and their practitioners exist only as processual and situated social relations. Choice architectures are neither stable and centred or fragmented and chaotic but restless and unpredictable, constantly becoming in situ and always in structuration. Only by approaching applied political theories in this way is it possible to understand disaster capitalism and neoliberalism redux on the one hand, and constitution of an Overton window on the other as contingent, original, and active accomplishments.

b. *Placing neoliberalism's metaphysical commitment to human freedom as non-interference at the heart of the UK's choice architectures and pandemic response*

At the heart of neoliberal logic is libertarianism and at the heart of libertarianism is the idea of freedom as non-interference. Arguably, it has been in and through this philosophy of human freedom that neoliberalism has most impacted the British government's pandemic response. Our approach contemplates the meaning and implications of thinking about freedom as non-interference and uses this reflection to better understand the aetiology of the narrow political imagination and self-limiting parameters that have underpinned the UK's public health response. Libertarian anxieties, aggravated by libertarian fundamentalists and lobbyists we argue, have actively produced a hesitant, reactive, insufficient, and at times counter-productive pandemic management strategy. We then explore the ways in which fidelity to freedom as non-interference has conspired to (a) denude the British state, weakening its institutions and capabilities; (b) place the figure of the autonomous market actor at the heart of British citizenship; and (c) widen inequalities and erode social cohesion and trust. In each case, our thesis is that neoliberalism has de facto waged a war of attrition on the UK's resilience and rendered the country susceptible to disproportionate harm from COVID-19.

Neoliberal political theory is grounded upon the pre-eminent value of individual freedom, in particular the "mercantile liberty" (Thorsen, 2010, 203) to trade, contract, and profit freely in the market as a sovereign economic agent. Such freedom, as a good in itself and as a means to human wellbeing, prosperity, and the efficient allocation of resources through market exchange (cf. Harvey, 2005, 2; Thorsen, 2010, 204), should therefore be protected and maximised as much as possible.

Importantly, neoliberals usually, though far from universally (see Irving, 2020), conceptualise freedom strictly as non-interference. For example, the leading neoliberal thinker, Milton Friedman, explicitly defined freedom as "the absence of coercion of one person by another" (1987, 7). This particular conception of freedom, famously categorised by Isaiah Berlin (1969) as 'negative liberty', views all interference qua interference as inimical to individual freedom. As such any and all interference by the state in the actions and choices of individuals—via coercive law, taxation, regulation, and so forth—represents a "tyrannical and oppressive" (Hall, 2011, 10) offense against freedom that must be minimised as much as possible, no matter how benign, paternalistic, or all-things-considered beneficial this interference may be.

Neoliberalism can therefore be seen to intersect closely with the libertarian tradition of contemporary political philosophy—in particular, the influential articulation of this tradition offered by Robert Nozick in his Anarchy, State, and Utopia (1974). Nozick argues that all humans are born with certain inalienable liberties and rights to self-ownership that mean they ought to be left in control of their own lives and free to do as they see fit (1974, 10). To protect these natural rights and liberties, the state must refrain from exerting undue interference or coercion that impinges on individuals' capacity to choose how best to live their lives. As Nozick argues: "Individuals have rights, and there are things no person or group may do to them (without violating their rights)...the state may not use its coercive apparatus for the purpose of getting some citizens to aid others, or in order to prohibit activities to people for their own good or protection" (1974, ix). As a case in point, Nozick offers the argument that "[t]axation of earnings from labor is on a par with forced labor" (1974, 169), claiming that redistributive taxation is equivalent to being compelled by the state to work for the good of someone else for free. Such coercion and interference, no matter how beneficent or paternalistic, erodes people's natural right to self-ownership and instead allows others (and the state itself) to treat them as a resource for the good of others. It fails to treat people as sovereign individuals who are responsible for their own choices and actions and free to decide how best to live their own lives.

Such a philosophical commitment to individual freedom as non-interference can be seen to have informed various strands of neoliberal policy and decision-making in the UK over recent decades, with policymakers seeking to minimise interference by the state in the lives of individuals as much as possible. In a 1968 Conservative Political Centre lecture, future Prime Minister, and Britain's first truly neoliberal leader, Margaret Thatcher, spelled out her understanding of freedom and its implications for public policy. Quoting John Stuart Mill, she defined freedom as "pursuing our own good in our own way" (Thatcher, 1968, 8), with government intervention believed to compromise freedom by reducing "the role of the individual, his importance and the desirability that he should be primarily responsible for his own future" (ibid., 7). This, Thatcher concluded, requires giving people "a far greater degree of personal responsibility and decision-making, far more independence from the government, and a comparative reduction in the role of government" (ibid., 5), including via reductions in the tax burden placed on individuals.

The tone was set. More generally, the neoliberal suspicion of state interference in people's lives, can be seen to underpin the idea of the 'nanny state', with the insinuation that government is an inherently patronising and constraining force in people's lives, which is abrogative of individual autonomy. This is an idea that seeks to discredit and de-legitimise the potential to use the democratic state as a means to protect the vulnerable and support people to flourish. In his book, *The Nanny State Made Me* (2020), the writer and broadcaster Stuart Maconie has recently documented how this corrosive narrative has taken hold of contemporary British discourse, normalised as a critique by the right-wing commentariat, and deployed by neoliberal policymakers to justify deregulation, privatisation, and the dismantling of the post-war welfare state. But what is so illiberal about an activist state? Is it always injurious to individual freedom? Can't state intervention also be liberating and emancipatory? As Maconie questions, "What was so terrible about properly funded hospitals, student grants, decent working conditions, affordable houses, trains that ran for convenience not profit, water that poured from the tap whose function was to slake your thirst not to make shareholders a dividend. What exactly was so wicked about public libraries, free eye tests and council houses?" (2020, x–xi).

The truth of course is that neoliberalism requires strong state intervention to prosper and there is nothing less Darwinian and more artificially constructed and socially engineered than a free market economy. Moreover, actually existing neoliberalism rarely presents as classical 'rollback' neoliberalism and is predicated upon state investment, albeit repurposed with particular goals in mind.

In the 1990s, for example, there emerged what might be referred to as state supplemented market fundamentalism. Drawing upon Anthony Gidden's (1998, 2000) theory of structuration and attempts to formulate a 'third way' between traditional Keynesianism and small state neoliberalism, Prime Minister Tony Blair's New Labour movement positioned itself as an antidote to neoliberal rule. In reality, the third way amounted to a form of rollout neoliberalism or better still a neoliberal governmentality designed to strengthen and cultivate the neoliberal subject and ergo the competitiveness of the UK economy in the context of a globalising and increasingly interconnected world. Thatcherite neoliberalism had failed to address the complex needs of communities debilitated by low aspiration, poverty, unemployment, family breakdown, poor housing, ill health, and low educational attainment. This loss of human potential was itself a drag on productivity and undermined the UK's global competitiveness. The role of the state was to invest in those communities left behind by rollback neoliberalism, but only so that they might be disciplined and responsibilised as competent market actors, consumers, and active citizens. The purpose of state intervention was to rehabilitate failing communities so that they could reproduce themselves autonomously and sustainably within the market economy. A convoluted apparatus of rewards and penalties—technes of neoliberal governmentality—was to impose moral norms concerning which forms of community were 'good' and 'bad'/'right' and 'wrong'/'just' and 'unjust'/'worthy' and 'unworthy'.

   c. *Reclaiming the idea of freedom from its neoliberal imprisonment and standing up an alternative political theory of freedom—in our case the neorepublican formulation of freedom as non-domination—as a counter-factual.*

In the UK, neoliberalism continues to be championed with an almost evangelical zeal and continues to capture—and to limit—the UK's political 'common sense'. For this reason, we have chosen to scope out a case for a renewed social democracy predicated on reclaiming freedom from its incarceration within the neoliberal dogma.

   Of course, there are many justifying logics for championing a renewed social democracy. We chose to use neorepublican theories of freedom so as to challenge the very basis of neoliberalism's claim that any return to significant state intervention—even if in the context of a pandemic event—constitutes a threat to long cherished liberal freedoms. The cure they say, must not be worse than the disease. We believe this supposition to be contrived and unwarranted. We too would wish to defend the values of human freedom, self-determination, entrepreneurship, and autonomy. But we believe that human freedom is best secured through social democratic capitalism and economic democracy and not liberal meritocratic capitalism and market fundamentalism. It is provincial and perverse to construe freedom and enhanced resilience as oppositional and antagonistic; in fact, if approached anew it is possible if not necessary to conceive of enhanced freedom as the very condition of possibility of fortified resilience. The cure will only be curative if is not also the cause of the disease!

   That the UK government has at times pitted its response as a balance between safeguarding freedoms, liberties, and human rights on the one hand and defending public safety and health on the other is perverse and injurious to both. Freedom, we contend, is not the enemy of public health, nor public health the enemy of freedom. In fact, one cannot prosper without the other. Although treated by advocates of neoliberalism as almost primordial, freedom as non-interference is but one idea of freedom; it is historically peculiar, politically produced, and congenitally parochial. It is an idea of freedom that rests upon suppositions which are far from innocent and which come freighted with vested interests and agendas. We too would wish to place a weight of importance on the value of individual liberty and work to protect this value through constitutional design and political decision-making. Freedom qua freedom remains a worthy root ideal upon which to build a better society. But evidently, conceptions of freedom are not made equally: some are more worthy than others and in the context of this book, some are better placed than others to save lives.

Drawing upon the neorepublican tradition of political philosophy, we contrast the idea of freedom as non-interference with an alternative formulation—freedom as non-domination. We revisit this dualism throughout this book, interrogating in each case the difference a gestalt switch might make. We chose this kind of recurrent normative narrative thread—as opposed to a final normative chapter—to better align and to reinforce—the counter-factual thought experiment we develop.

IMPLICATIONS OF OUR CHOSEN METHODOLOGICAL STRATEGY

Our methodological strategy—applied political theory—has implications for the way we think about each of diagnosis (why has the UK government failed the COVID-19 test?), panacea (what does the UK government need to fix if it is to 'fail forward'?), prescription (how might the UK government fix what needs to be fixed?), and prognoses (how likely is that the UK government will in fact build back better?). We offer four central propositions:

- **Diagnoses**: The UK government's root politico-economic-institutional model—its commitment to neoliberal freedoms and market fundamentalism—lies at the heart of the country's heightened vulnerability, elevated susceptibility to harm, and shocking COVID-19 death rates.
- **Panacea**: COVID-19 has brought us to a pivot point in history: nothing less than a new political dispensation/social compact will

be required if the UK is to authentically fortify its resilience in preparation for future pandemics and other shock events.

- **Prescription**: We need to provincialise the neoliberal capture of the idea of 'freedom' and stand up a better alternative. The neorepublican tradition of political philosophy has fashioned a superior concept of freedom that recasts freedom as constitutive of—and indeed constituted by—social democracy and not its antithesis.
- **Prognosis**: Neoliberalism redux is a powerful force but COVID-19 has further weakened the UK's already crisis prone neoliberal model and has triggered a fresh structuration of this model. The extent to which there exists worldly politics capable of enacting a new social compact remains a live puzzle.

Let us now unpack each argument in turn.

Diagnosis: Why Has the UK Failed the COVID-19 Test?

Globally, the translation of theoretical or proto-neoliberalism into actually existing neoliberalism betrays a long and colourful history. We pick up this story in the late 1970s and early 1980s when, following the collapse of the Fordist-Keynesian compromise, the Thatcher government introduced neoliberalism as the guiding normative theory for the UK state. In the decades which followed, the UK has become one of the world's furthest, fastest, and most enthusiastic converts to the neoliberal political programme; indeed, the country has become something of a poster child for neoliberal reform. Neoliberalism has become ingrained as the common sense or received wisdom of the UK state and now naturalises what are in fact highly political choice architectures. So omnipresent are neoliberal assumptions in the reflexive instincts of policymakers that the pithy slogan 'there is no alternative' has become a literal truism.

Our core provocation is that the COVID-19 pandemic has cruelly exposed the failings of the neoliberal system which has proven an inadequate and actively harmful foundation for state governance of crises. Successive UK governments have presided over a degeneration of social democracy and sponsored a socio-political formation which is no longer supportive of human flourishing. Indeed, in our view neoliberalism has proven to be actively harmful to the public health response (indeed, it has created something of a hostile environment for effective public health interventions) and has itself amplified an already dangerous pandemic into a national disaster. In pursuit of a sectarian idea of freedom, neoliberalism has broken the social compact between the government and the citizenry. As the United Nations Special Rapporteur on extreme poverty and human rights Philip Alston commented presciently following a visit to the UK in 2019: "The bottom line is that much of the glue that has held British society together since the Second World War has been deliberately removed and replaced with a harsh and uncaring ethos". Without such a compact it is impossible to conceive of, let alone enact, an impactful public health response to the pandemic. It is here that we must surely start if we are to properly understand the toll COVID-19 has exacted on the UK.

We examine the impact of various logics and legacies that stem from neoliberal theories of freedom—*freedom as non-interference*—on key progenitors of poor outcomes. By logics we refer to the ingrained philosophical commitments, norms, and assumptions, rooted in neoliberal political theory, that have come to inform government decision-making in the contemporary UK. Legacies, on the other hand, refer to the long-term social and economic impacts of these logics playing out through policymaking. The net effect of these logics and legacies, we show, has been to severely hamper the UK's resilience and response to the COVID-19 pandemic, leading to a hesitant, often chaotic, approach to the crisis and one that has rarely aligned with international best practice. For illustration, we will examine the impact of neoliberal reform on each of the state, the citizen, and socio-spatial inequalities, showing how market fundamentalism has denuded each, creating in its wake: (a) a state that has been slow and less responsive in its responsibilities, (b) atomised neoliberal citizen-subjects who privilege self-reliance over social solidarity, and (c) ever widening wealth and income inequalities (Table 1.1).

Panacea: What Does the UK Government Need to Fix If It Is to 'Fail Forward'?

As we seek to build back better from the pandemic, we must recognise that the neoliberal model is on critical life support and is no longer fit for purpose. Given the comparative failure of the UK's neoliberal polity to respond adequately to the COVID-19 crisis, the foundations for post-pandemic renewal, categorically, cannot be neoliberal. Better public

Table 1.1 Neoliberal logics and legacies and the *production* of vulnerability to COVID-19 in the UK

Neoliberal freedom: Freedom as non-interference, or freedom from any and all coercion and constraint

Neoliberal freedom and the denudation of the UK state

Logics	Only a minimal state can be justified; other than to prop up the market and lubricate its functioning, neoliberals are unwilling to expand the roles and responsibilities of the state
Legacies	*Before COVID-19:* shrinking of the state, and its roles and responsibilities, e.g. through privatisation, arms-length industrial strategy, austerity cuts to the public realm, etc
	During COVID-19: emphasis on market solutions to the pandemic, e.g. public–private partnerships to deliver test and trace capacity. State intervention and abnormal aberration to be reversed at the first opportunity, not a pivot towards a revived Keynesianism

Neoliberal freedom and the denudation of the active citizen in the UK

Logics	Emphasis on personal responsibility, suspicion of democracy. If it is the market where we exercise our freedom, express our agency, and generate social good, what need do we have for expansive democratic politics?
Legacies	*Before COVID-19:* a "great risk shift" with increasing precarity for citizens and erosion of collective safety net. Depoliticisation of decision-making, e.g. Bank of England independence. And weakening of civic engagement, e.g. declining voter turnout
	During COVID-19: emphasis on personal, rather than collective, responsibility to combat the virus. "Depoliticisation" of decision making ("guided by the science"). Aversion to democratic scrutiny

Neoliberal freedom, the denudation of social justice, and growing inequalities in the UK.

Logics	Whatever arises from the application of just steps is itself just, whilst interventions to alleviate inequalities pose a threat to liberty
Legacies	*Before COVID-19:* widening inequalities in health, wealth, and prosperity. Worsening health outcomes following a social gradient.
	During COVID-19: pandemic has exploited and exacerbated existing inequalities, disproportionately impacting UK's most disadvantaged communities

Source Authors own

policy choices can, of course, always be made within the existing politico-economic-institutional model. But to double down on the norms, logics, and approaches of neoliberalism now would only serve to rebuild a political order that has been shown to be practically, as well as ethically, unsound—potentially leaving the UK population as at risk from further communicable diseases and, indeed, other external shocks, as it was from COVID-19. We will make insufficient progress if we simply medicate ourselves on a barely modified status quo.

Prescription: How Might the UK Government Fix What Needs to Be Fixed?

Neoliberalism's hegemonic, though partial and subjective, concept of freedom lies at the heart of the UK's difficulties. It has been used (and misused) to, both implicitly and explicitly, constrain, guide, and structure the UK government's decision-making through the course of the pandemic. We must constantly remind ourselves that the idea of freedom per se is a critically important one; the problem is not freedom itself but instead its interpretation, capture, and appropriation by neoliberalism. For us, this means reclaiming freedom which has been hijacked by neoliberalism and rendered simply as *non-interference* and putting an alternative neorepublican idea of 'just freedom' or *freedom as non-domination* in the service of a new social democratic compact and a build back better project which is genuinely disruptive and transformative. The neorepublican tradition offers a theory of freedom that is congruous with social democracy—indeed that understands social democracy to be the essential guarantor of freedom and freedom a prerequisite for a healthy social democracy.

We elaborate this proposal throughout the book, pointing to the ways in which—viewed through a neorepublican prism, social democracy supports rather than diminishes human freedom whilst expanding human freedom invigorates rather than erodes social solidarity. We argue that idea of freedom as non-domination opens up very different ways of thinking about the state, the citizen, and inequalities in democratic politics, and provides normative justification for a broader range of policy responses in the face of crises such as the COVID-19 pandemic (Table 1.2).

Table 1.2 Schematic summary of key ideas in Neoliberal and Neorepublican thought as they bear on the argument arc of this book

	Neoliberal thought	Neorepublican thought
Key thinkers and their works	Friedrich Hayek, *The Road to Serfdom* (1944) Milton Friedman, *Capitalism and Freedom* (1962) Robert Nozick, *Anarchy, State, and Utopia* (1974)	Philip Pettit, *Republicanism: A Theory of Freedom and Government* (1997) Quentin Skinner, *Liberty Before Liberalism* (2012 [1998]) Frank Lovett, *A General Theory of Domination and Justice* (2010)
Anchor concept of freedom	*Freedom as non-interference*, or freedom from any and all coercion and constraint	*Freedom as non-domination*, or freedom from arbitrary interference only
Implications of/for *The role of the state*	**Neoliberal freedom** Only a minimal ('rolled back') state can be justified, one which limits its intervention in the market and in people's lives as much as possible. In reality considerable state effort is expended supporting the market to function ('roll out' neoliberalism)	**Neorepublican freedom** A suitably republican (for us social democratic) state can intervene to combat sources of domination that may arise in society and promote the common good
The role of the citizen	Denuded conception of citizenship—neoliberal subjects are expected to accept personal responsibility for their lives and express preferences through the market. Democratic participation is devalorised with emphasis placed on 'depoliticised' technocracy	Vigilant, contestatory forms of participatory democracy and democratic citizenship are necessary to ensure government interventions are non-arbitrary and compatible with freedom

(continued)

Table 1.2 (continued)

	Neoliberal thought	Neorepublican thought
The causes and remediation of inequalities	The market leads to growth overall, and over time social justice and equity ('trickle down'). Socioeconomic disparity (to the extent that they persist) can be dismissed by neoliberals as both an acceptable outcome of free exchange, and beyond the purview of legitimate state intervention in the lives of free individuals	Freedom prospers only in the context of intersubjective equality. It is the responsibility of a suitably republican state to maintain protective, regulatory, and empowering institutions that enable individuals to interact as free and equal citizens. Liberty means nothing unless it is supported by equality of opportunity

Source Author's own

Prognoses: How Likely Is That the UK Government Will in Fact Build Back Better?

During its brief existence, the neoliberal regime has accumulated an impressive résumé of socially painful crises. Forty years of market fundamentalism has sculpted an economy that not only has registered at best mediocre growth rates but which has lurched from one crisis to the next, creating endless and socially painful cycles of boom and bust. Climate change, widening inequalities, nationalistic populist movements, and a mental health crisis are bringing an already precarious neoliberal model to the brink. And into this volatile mix has come COVID-19. The latest shock. In consequence, it is hardly surprising that social consent for the model has been depleted to the extent that some critics now believe it to be in its end times. It is not altogether fanciful to suppose that COVID-19 could in time join the pantheon of episodes when communicable diseases have served as hinge points in the unfolding of history: the catalyst of a speeding up of the collapse of the past. Perhaps in future we will come to recognise this moment as a hinge point in history, when the global pandemic proved to be the straw that finally broke neoliberalism and when the green shoots of a new social democratic regulatory regime first entered the world.

But this is to get ahead of ourselves.

A signature if puzzling feature of neoliberalism is its 'Houdini-like' ability to exploit crises—including those that it was centrally implicated in creating—first by spawning an emergency disaster capitalism and secondly but offering an even more aggressively neoliberal post-crash regulatory environment as the only solution. Certainly, the UK's COVID-19 regulatory institutions and experiments and its nascent post-pandemic politico-institutional architecture and growth agenda do not signal that a moment of genuine disruption and reset is imminent. Disaster capitalism and neoliberalism redux are once again threatening to foreclose possibilities. In spite of protestations about the inadequacy of the status quo, 'build back better' projects are already wearing the clothes of 'business as usual'. *Plus ça change, plus c'est la même chose?*

But again, this is to get ahead of ourselves.

In reality, this is a moment when agonising losses and hard-fought victories will combine one way or another to bring newness into the world. This might in the end lead to a transmogrification and eclipsing of the neoliberal order. It might however simply birth a new generation of disaster capitalism, further accumulation by dispossession and consolidate neoliberalism redux. And so, we are led to ask a question that lies at the bottom of it all; what impact will the pandemic itself have on the odyssey of the UK's neoliberal project and indeed the neoliberal experiment more broadly? Whatever happens, newness will enter the world. The precise trajectory of British neoliberalism will be a contingent outcome of place-based political contestation, struggles over regulatory reform, and the contextual and contingent structuration of neoliberal institutions. In this we must not confuse any apparent post-pandemic neoliberalism redux as a simple reset after a shock or a blip; if it happens it needs to be viewed as an active, historically novel, and ultimately vulnerable reinvention and reimagining. The future will need to be made and it will be made variously over space, further complexifying actually existing neoliberalism's complex geographies.

A Guide to the Structure of the Chapters to Follow

In Chapter 2, we elaborate our approach and introduce the intellectual resources we will deploy to render intelligible neoliberalism as a coherent tradition within contemporary political thought and the imbrication of neoliberalism in the UK's encounter with COVID-19 and COVID-19 in the structuration of the UK's neoliberal project. In Chapter 3 we ask; just how poorly has the UK performed and on the basis of which metrics?

In Chapters 4–7, we expose the corrosive impact of neoliberalism on the UK's resilience to near perpetual crisis in the opening decades of the twenty-first century. In Chapter 4, we set the scene by focussing upon the ways in which the neoliberal capture of the idea of freedom as non-interference has been pivotal in shaping the UK's response. We introduce the alternative neorepublican idea of freedom as non-domination to provincialise neoliberalism's capture of 'freedom' and to underscore how, if approached anew, it is possible to reimagine the nexus between freedom and social democracy as mutually enriching and the basis for a more resilient UK and efficacious UK government pandemic response. We build this case across the next three chapters which combine analytical and normative reasoning to explore inter-alia the themes of state, citizen, and inequality. Each chapter considers how these concepts are understood within neoliberal thought (the logics), and how these theories have informed UK policymaking over recent decades (the legacies).

In each of these sections, we show how a plausible alternative, derived from republican political theory, could have supported a very different approach to the pandemic by UK policymakers.

We conclude (Chapter 8) with the claim that in recovery, the UK must now break away from simply reheating the (notably protean) neoliberal paradigm. To meaningfully 'build back better' a true renaissance of social democracy is needed, not just a neoliberal imitation that can only ever offer piecemeal and tokenistic reform. For those who consider that political philosophy begins and ends with the idea of human freedom, we offer neorepublican thought as a coherent intellectual alternative to neoliberalism and call upon the idea of freedom as non-domination in the service of rebuilding British social democracy for enhanced resilience.

CONCLUSION

Pandemics of plague, smallpox, cholera, influenza, polio, measles, malaria, and typhus have played a crucial role in shaping the fortunes and fate of many past human civilizations. It is not altogether fanciful to suppose that COVID-19 could in time join the pantheon of episodes when communicable diseases have served as hinge points in the unfolding of big history. COVID-19 is a barometer of sorts for the UK, and 'the West', revealing its vulnerabilities and surfacing ongoing weaknesses and deficiencies in its already-faltering civilizational model. Perhaps it might even prove in the end to be one crisis too many, the nudge that will finally topple the house of cards in this age of perma-crisis. In COVID-19, we might just be witnessing a speeding-up of the collapse of the past.

REFERENCES

Berlin, I. (1969). *Four essays on liberty*. Oxford University Press.
Friedman, M. (1987). Free markets and free speech. *Harvard Journal of Law and Public Policy, 10*(1), 1–10.
Giddens, A. (1998). *The third way: The renewal of social democracy*. Polity.
Giddens, A. (2000). *The third way and its critics*. Polity.
Giroux, H. A. (2021). The Covid-19 Pandemic is exposing the plague of neoliberalism. In N. K. Denzin and M. D. Giardina (Eds.), *Collaborative futures in qualitative inquiry research in a pandemic*, 17–26. Routledge.

Glover, R. E., & Maani, N. (2020). Have we reached "peak neoliberalism" in the UK's covid-19 response? https://blogs.bmj.com/bmj/2021/01/27/have-we-reached-peak-neoliberalism-in-the-uks-covid-19-response/. Accessed 28 Dec 2021.

Hall, S. (2011). The neoliberal revolution. *Soundings, 48,* 9–27.

Harvey, D. (2005). *A brief history of neoliberalism.* Oxford University Press.

Health and Social Care and Science and Technology Committees. (2021). *Coronavirus: Lessons learned to date* (HC 2021–22, 92). House of Commons.

Horton, R. (2021). *The COVID-19 catastrophe: What's gone wrong and how to stop it happening again.* John Wiley & Sons.

Irving, S. (2020). Hayek's neo-Roman liberalism. *European Journal of Political Theory, 19*(4), 553–570.

Maconie, S. (2020). *The Nanny state made me.* Ebury Press.

Mellish, T. I., Luzmore, N. J., & Shahbaz, A. A. (2020). Why were the UK and USA unprepared for the COVID-19 pandemic? The systemic weaknesses of neoliberalism: A comparison between the UK, USA, Germany, and South Korea. *Journal of Global Faultlines, 7*(1), 9–45.

Navarro, V. (2020). The consequences of neoliberalism in the current pandemic. *International Journal of Health Services, 50*(3), 271–275.

Nozick, R. (1974). *Anarchy, state, and utopia.* Blackwell.

Rancière, J. (2004). *The politics of aesthetics: The distribution of the sensible.* Continuum London.

Saad-Filho, A. (2020). From COVID-19 to the end of neoliberalism. *Critical Sociology, 46,* 477–485.

Smith, N. (2006). There's no such thing as a natural disaster. https://items.ssrc.org/understanding-katrina/theres-no-such-thing-as-a-natural-disaster/. Accessed 28 Dec 2021.

Sparke, M., & Williams, O. D. (2022). Neoliberal disease: COVID-19, co-pathogenesis and global health insecurities. *Environment and Planning A: Economy and Space, 54*(1), 15–32.

Standring, A., & Davies, J. (2020). From crisis to catastrophe: The death and viral legacies of austere neoliberalism in Europe? *Dialogues in Human Geography, 10*(2), 146–149.

Sultana, F. (2021). Climate change, COVID-19, and the co-production of injustices: A feminist reading of overlapping crises. *Social & Cultural Geography, 22*(4), 447–460.

Šumonja, M. (2021). Neoliberalism is not dead–On political implications of Covid-19. *Capital & Class, 45*(2), 215–227.

Thatcher, M. (1968). Conservative political centre (CPC) lecture ("what's wrong with politics?"). https://www.margaretthatcher.org/document/101632. Accessed 28 Dec 2021.

Thorsen, D. E. (2010). The neoliberal challenge: What is neoliberalism? *Contemporary Readings in Law and Social Justice, 2*(2), 188–214.

CHAPTER 2

A Brief Introduction to the Odyssey of (British) Neoliberalism

Abstract Our argument is that the UK's deleterious encounter with COVID-19 needs to be understood as an outworking of the nexus between a failing British neoliberal model and a historically exceptional pandemic event. However, before getting to COVID-19, we must take a step back and consider first the odyssey of market fundamentalism and the trajectory and travails of British neoliberalism. And, to do this, we must take a second step back and reflect critically upon how we might define and conceptualise neoliberalism and narrate the story of its manifestations, embeddings, and mutations in the institutional context of the UK.

Keywords Neoliberalism · Market fundamentalism · Neoliberalism redux · Freedom as non-interference · Political economy · Build back better

INTRODUCTION

Our argument is that the UK's deleterious encounter with COVID-19 needs to be understood as an outworking of the nexus between a failing British neoliberal model and a historically exceptional pandemic event. However, before getting to COVID-19, we must take a step back and

© The Author(s), under exclusive license to Springer Nature Switzerland AG 2022
M. Boyle et al., *COVID-19 and the Case Against Neoliberalism*,
https://doi.org/10.1007/978-3-031-18935-7_2

consider first the odyssey of market fundamentalism and the trajectory and travails of British neoliberalism. To do this, we must take a second step back and reflect critically upon how we might define and conceptualise neoliberalism and narrate the story of its manifestations, embeddings, and mutations in the institutional context of the UK.

In his recent paper, *Confessions of a recovering régulation theorist*, Jamie Peck (2022) reflects upon the importance of the rise, reign, and faltering of Parisian regulation theory in the development of scholarly interest in the rise, reign, and faltering of neoliberalism, not least in the US and the UK over the past forty years. For Peck, in the 1980s, at a time when political forces appeared to be blowing in a new, consequential, and for some worrying direction, regulation theory provided a helpful if rigid schematic for periodising past political-economic compacts and making sense of what appeared to be a renewed interest in market fundamentalism. But it soon became painfully obvious that the school's ontology—resting as it did on the possibility of the existence of stable regimes of accumulation albeit interspersed with moments of rupture and spasm—was deeply flawed. Neoliberalism by its nature was crisis prone and the idea that it might ever reach a steady state equilibrium was misconceived. Moreover neoliberalism was more a *modality* of regulation than a *mode* of regulation; there was no such thing as proto-neoliberalism or pristine neoliberalism, only ever actually existing neoliberalism or better still only ever contextual, contingent, and contested *neoliberalisation*. Neoliberalism has to be understood as an unpredictable and emergent *process*; pro-market institutional redesign, toiling on an inherited social democratic institutional landscape, resulting in a messy amalgam of hybrid, provisional and transitory institutional experiments. Neoliberalism is always in mutation and never simply in maturation; it is never stable, always restless and fluid; never a settled institutional compact but always in structuration; never a fixture, always a fixation; and never in fossilised stasis, always adapting to crises and shape shifting. And to make matters more complex again, all of this doing, undoing, and redoing of regulatory infrastructure, necessarily plays out variously over space and time.

Peck concludes that whilst a key milestone in the theorisation of capitalist regulation, scholarship on the regulation of neoliberalism has necessarily progressed beyond the strictures of regulation theory, at least its early formulations.

Aside from finding it insightful, we will use Peck's *Confessions* article somewhat imaginatively here as *method:* a technique for sequencing an accessible entrée to British neoliberalism. We begin this chapter then by harnessing Parisian regulation theory, or at least its most essential ideas, to provide a rudimentary orientation to the story of the ascent of British neoliberalism. Suspending nuance and complexity and cautioning that a more sophisticated elaboration will follow, we aim here simply to provide the reader with a basic anchoring narrative arc. We then note that whilst powerful, the term neoliberalism comes freighted with troubling controversies, complications, and confusions; so much so that some scholars now advocate its abandonment *tout court*. We interrogate calls for its banishment from the academy and make a counter case for its preservation as an indispensable analytic resource for the times in which we live. On this basis, and informed by Peck's theoretical agenda, we finally clarify how we will be putting the specific idea of *neoliberalism as process* to work in the remainder of this book.

The Odyssey of (British) Neoliberalism

Published in 1976 as a book titled *A Theory of Capitalist Regulation: The US Experience*, Michel Aglietta's monumental study of the trajectory of the US economy from the Civil War of the early 1860s to Jimmy Carter's election as US President in 1976 has come to be viewed as the seminal text in the Parisian Regulation School (l'école de la régulation). Aglietta asks; given that capitalism has an innate tendency towards crisis, why has it survived over time and managed to endure? What makes capitalism so resilient given its manifest capacity to go awry?

For Aglietta at any given point in time there exists a dominant 'regime of accumulation': a particular structure, pattern, and order to the production and consumption of commodities. Left to their own devices, regimes of accumulation are unlikely to survive very long. What allows them to be sustained, at least for a period, is the existence of parallel 'modes of regulation'; formal and informal institutions which prop up given systems of production and consumption and afford them technical efficacy and social legitimacy. But contradictions in the system can only be suspended for a window of time. When regulation fails, the prevailing politico-economic model defaults and a crisis arises. Crises could of course persist endlessly as the new norm; the alternative is that a new regime of accumulation and mode of regulation emerge from the struggle to 'build back better', enabling a new tradition of capitalism to prosper for another epoch.

According to Aglietta, the history of capitalism then, can be construed as a cycle, with periods of stability and growth punctuated by periods of crises—or more accurately periods of crises interspersed with moments of deferred crises. For most of the period up until the First World War including and in particular the Victorian Era, and thereafter the 'roaring (19)20s', laissez-faire free market capitalism became the central pillar of economic policy. German Philosopher Karl Marx referred to this period as the age of 'vulgar capitalism': Darwinian survival of the fittest reigned. An interesting counter-factual is provided by periods in the twentieth century (the First and Second World Wars, and a Keynesian moment between 1945 and 1975) when the application of market rule was less disciplined and social democratic logic and state economic management prevailed. Nonetheless, the past forty years have witnessed the rise once again of neoliberal economic orthodoxies and a rekindling of interest in small state, low taxation, liberalised free markets, privatism, deregulation, and entrepreneurial freedoms.

Let us now apply this framework to discern in greater detail the historical context in which neoliberalism emerged and took shape.

The Fordist-Keynesian Compromise: Les Trente Glorieuses (1945–1973)

From the 1880s onwards, and guided by US mechanical engineer Frederick Taylor, there emerged in the western world a tradition of applied scholarship called Scientific Management (Taylor, 1911). Scientific Management placed under scrutiny the working practices of industries and factories with a view to making those practices more reliable, efficient, and productive. It was in this climate that US industrialist Henry Ford began to examine critically the methods through which automobiles were being produced. Ford established a car production plant in Detroit, Michigan, and in this plant pioneered two notable innovations, the division of labour and the assembly line. The result of these changes was a quantum increase in worker productivity and the advent mass production. Ford recognised that the sustainability of his firm was dependent upon worker loyalty and the existence of a market for his cars. He solved both in part by offering workers pay increases in line with improvements in productivity.

Ford's approach to production came to be copied by manufacturers in many industries, in the US and subsequently throughout the industrial world. By World War II, Fordist mass production was assumed to hold the key to economic growth and prosperity. But Ford's interest in building employee loyalty, securing peaceable labour relations, and ensuring the existence of a market for mass-produced goods presented a challenge to governments. Firms could not solve this problem by themselves; a structural solution across the entire economy was needed.

In searching for such a solution many governments turned to the ideas of British economist John Maynard Keynes. Keynes wrote his seminal book *The General Theory of Employment, Interest and Money* in 1936 during the Great Depression when unemployment grew to as much as 30% in many countries (unemployment was as high as 25% in the US). The market, Keynes famously declared, could remain irrational longer than people could stay solvent; markets were moved by 'animal spirits' and not 'reason'. Capitalism was based on 'the extraordinary belief that the nastiest of men for the nastiest of motives will somehow work together for the benefit of all'. State regulation was essential. But what type of regulation was required? For Keynes aggregate demand in the economy was key. As long as there were buyers there would be sellers, as long as there were sellers there would be employment, and as long as there were workers there would be consumer demand. In conditions of market failure, it was the job of the government to inject demand into the economy; to spend more even when spending less appears to be more logical.

The extent to which Keynes' ideas had any impact upon President Franklin D. Roosevelt's New Deal (1933–1939) and massive public work programme remains the subject of debate. But certainly after WW2, inspired by Keynes' theory of demand-led economic growth, many governments around the world—including in the United Kingdom—entered into social partnerships with Fordist firms and labour and trade union movements. Partnerships, collective agreements, and social contracts were forged. Workers would receive pay rises pegged to productivity improvements. The higher the productivity of the labour force the greater the remuneration. Also, governments established welfare states. Through general taxation, workers would be provided with social protection (such as unemployment benefits and pensions) and items of collective consumption, such as health care, education, and housing. Productivity increases would guarantee better protection and more services.

This marriage between the political system and the economy came to be known as the Fordist-Keynesian compromise. Using the language of the regulation school, we may say that Fordism emerged as the principal regime of accumulation whilst the Keynesian welfare state, its mode of regulation. Between 1945 and 1975 this compromise led to historically unrivalled economic growth, prosperity, and improved standards of living throughout the Western world. This period is now referred to as the thirty glory years of capitalism (per regulation theory, *les trente glorieuses*).

But by the mid-1970s, the Fordist-Keynesian compromise began to come unstuck. In part, problems were caused by a number of external shocks to the capitalist world, including a series of wars and oil crises. In particular, the decision in 1973 by the Organization of Petroleum Exporting Countries (OPEC) to quadruple the price of oil in protest over western support for Israel during the Yom Kippur War was followed by a second oil crisis in 1979 when the price of oil doubled as the Iranian Revolution unfolded. Combined with the economic impacts of the Vietnam War (1955–1975), these hikes caused a profit squeeze in the West's oil-fired economies and led to economic turbulence.

But in fact, by the late 1960s and the early 1970s, the system itself was in crisis. External shocks merely toppled a regime of accumulation that was already structurally compromised (Piore & Sabel, 1984). Scientific Management and Fordism had squeezed out of production processes and systems all of the productivity gains that were possible. Annual increases in production across the economy began to wane and the law of diminishing returns set in. But social partnerships remained strong and the labour movement continued to demand more wages and governments more taxation. Having enjoyed thirty years of expansion, neither were minded to enter into a new relationship with the capitalist economy. There were to be no new renegotiated deals between firms, workers, and governments. It proved politically impossible to curb demands for wage inflation and continuous expansion of welfare states. Firms simply had to subsidise both. With costs increasing as before but productivity increases stalling and output stabilising, firms found themselves unable to maintain their profit margins and their rate of profit decreased. Thrashing to reverse this squeeze upon their profitability and capacity to pay dividends to shareholders, they conspired to plunge the entire system into crisis. A new international division of labour emptied the advanced capitalist world of swathes of manufacturing capacity.

Neoliberalism: On the Hidden Hand of the Market

In his classic works *The Theory of Moral Sentiments* (1758) and *An Inquiry into the Nature and Causes of the Wealth of Nations* (1776), Scottish economist and philosopher Adam Smith famously argued that self-interest and laissez-faire open and free markets operate not only to grow wealth overall but also to distribute that wealth so that it enhances the welfare of all peoples in all places. The 'hidden-hand of the market' not only referred to the inbuilt capacity of markets to maximise economic efficiency, it also referred to the market's inbuilt capacity to administer moral sentiment. Elaborated, reworked, and further propagated over the next 250 years by a wide variety of classical and neoclassical economists, much has been claimed for—and expected of—Smith's thesis and its apotheosis, globalising liberalised free market capitalism.

In 1944, Austrian-British economist and philosopher Friedrich August von Hayek published a book titled *The Road to Serfdom* in which he first articulated the theoretical principles on 'neoliberalism'—this lab-based thought experiment was to be labelled proto-type neoliberalism or proto-neoliberalism. Disaffected by worrying political developments in European countries, Hayek condemned the tyranny of fascism and socialism, and in particular the rise of National Socialism in Germany. Centrally planned economies had a proclivity to degenerate into dictatorial economies, he argued. The solution was limited government and radically laissez-faire capitalism. In 1947, thirty-six economists, historians, and philosophers met at the invitation of Hayek at Mont Pelerin in Switzerland, after which an influential neoliberal advocacy group—the Mont Pelerin Society—was born. Hayek was to move to the University of Chicago where he inspired American fellow economist and statistician Milton Friedman, also a proponent of free market capitalism. In his 1962 book, Capitalism and Freedom, Friedman, rejected the prevailing Keynesian approach (demand management) to economic management preferring instead Monetarist policies (or supply side economics).

It was not until the late 1970s and the crash of the Fordist-Keynesian model that Hayek and Friedmann's neoliberal ideas were to move from the fringe to centre stage. The propagation of the ideology of neoliberalism, betrays a long and colourful history. The 'Chicago Boys', a label applied to a collection of Chilean economists who were trained at the Department of Economics of the University of Chicago under the tutelage of Friedman in the 1970s and 1980s, returned to Chile with neoliberal ideas; at the behest of General Augusto Pinochet (Chile's dictator who ruled from 1973 to 1990) these ideas were applied, seemingly at first blush with positive results. Neoliberalism crashed onto the shores of both the UK and the US in the 1980s in the guise of Thatcherism and Reaganism. It became the dominant ideology proffered by the 'holy trinity': the World Bank, IMF, and WTO, who sought to build a 'Washington consensus' which decreed that neoliberalism was the only economic model capable of lifting Global South countries out of poverty. Neoliberal Structural Adjustment Programmes were exported to and imposed upon bankrupt nations as a condition of bailout loans.

From 1979 to the present day, more generally, neoliberalism has replaced Fordist-Keynesianism as the dominant economic model in many western core countries. As firms have strived to restore profitability, a war has been waged on organised labour movements and welfare states, both of which have found themselves weakened and disempowered. According to David Harvey (2005) a new era of neoliberal capitalism has developed in which capitalist firms have freed themselves from 'burdens' imposed upon them during the Fordist-Keynesian period. To be competitive in the global economy firms need to be entrepreneurial, lean, mean, and flexible. For this to happen, it is argued, workers need to offer their labour at cheaper rates and be prepared to accept flexible terms and conditions. It also requires, it is contended, that governments reduce taxation and downsize welfare states. But neoliberal capitalism has created a volatile and unstable world and has yet to discover a formula as successful as the Fordist-Keynesian compromise. The law of the jungle has set in; in the struggle for survival only the leanest and meanest can make it.

Of course, caution is due as the origins, dispersal, and penetration of neoliberal ideas have been uneven and contested. Danish Sociologist Gøsta Esping-Andersen (1990) identified the UK (alongside the US) as paradigmatic of liberal capitalism and contrasted this model with corporatist statist capitalism (whose iconic example was Germany) and social democratic capitalism (embodied by the Nordic states). In a similar vein, the European studies scholar Peter Hall and British economist David Soskice (2001) have called for more attention to be given to varieties of capitalism (VoC) and have distinguished therein between liberal market economies (the Anglo-Saxon countries of the US, the UK, Canada, Australia, New Zealand, Ireland) and coordinated market economies (for example, the Nordics and other European countries such as Germany, Belgium, the Netherlands, and Austria). More broadly, Serbian-American

Economist Branko Milanovic (2019) differentiates two types of capitalism: the 'liberal meritocratic capitalism' of the West (again the US and UK present as iconic examples), and the 'state-led political, or authoritarian, capitalism' that has fuelled the rise of South-East Asia.

Although the power of the 'unleashed' market has led to impressive growth in some places, in fact generally economic growth rates under neoliberalism have been inferior to those achieved under the Fordist-Keynesian model. But returns to societies' elites by contrast have been spectacular. According to Harvey (2007) the neoliberal capture of capitalism's regulatory apparatus, can be read as a decisive development in the class war over the division of the national product—an overt elite ideological project. For Harvey, neoliberalism is a political-economic project orchestrated by the top 1% for the top 1% (or at best top 10%) at the expense of the comparative wealth and income accrued by the bottom 50% and especially the bottom 10%.

Through what Harvey (2003) calls 'accumulation by dispossession', capital has reversed the gains to labour which were ushered in with the Fordist-Keynesian state and rising wages and restored inequalities in wealth back to Victorian levels. Rereading German economist, philosopher, and revolutionary Karl Marx's *Capital Volume 1: A Critique of Political Economy* (first published in 1867), Harvey drew parallels between neoliberalism and what Marx called 'original or primitive accumulation'; the dispossession by Europe of capital in the colonies through imperialism. Only now this dispossession was visiting economic injustices upon workers living in core countries who were being divested by four processes:

- Public assets, resources, property, and infrastructure have been privatised and commodified; this loss of public goods has benefitted a small number of private interests.
- Financial services (banks, insurance companies, pension and investment funds, and so on) have been deregulated inducing practices which, whilst having the potential of yielding huge profits, have also proven risky and at times reckless. Private actors accepted the profit whilst the public absorbed the risk.
- Through what has been termed 'disaster capitalism', powerful private interests have created and exploited economic crisis to secure 'vulture' profits; meanwhile, ordinary citizens have had to live with the carnage.

- The fiscal policies of neoliberal governments have persistently favoured actions which lubricate the market over those designed to redistribute wealth to those most in need.

Having lived through half a century of improving living standards and expanding government expenditure, both organised labour movements and welfare states have found it difficult to accept the collapse of social partnerships and attacks on wage increases, social entitlements, workers' rights, and public services. According to Harvey (2010), workers have sought to weather the vagaries and vicissitudes of neoliberal capitalism by borrowing from financial institutions and entering into debt. Expectations of continuous rises in standards of living were to be serviced only through borrowing and indebtedness. Keen to raise capital to lend to this growing market of borrowers, financial institutions have borrowed from other financial institutions, creating in turn a deeply interconnected global financial system. But the debt being accumulated is vast and servicing it is going to be a challenge. In 2008, financial institutions woke up to the realisation of just how vulnerable they were to debt default. A global meltdown of the financial system resulted, in turn bringing the global economy to its knees and catalysing a decade of savage austerity and painful structural adjustment across the capitalist world (Peck & Theodore, 2019). For all the talk of build back better, the past decade has witnessed (ever more) disaster capitalism and neoliberalism redux.

APPROACHING NEOLIBERALISM AS A CONTEXTUAL, CONTINGENT, AND CONTESTED PROCESS

We have written the above regulation theory inspired chronology to help the reader navigate through the arguments we make in the remainder of the book. Haunting our account has been a simple question that we have chosen to defer until now: but what exactly is neoliberalism! For us, neoliberalism, broadly speaking, describes a coherent and distinctive tradition of thought that draws on a range of normative ideas about politics, society, and economics from classical liberal and libertarian traditions. At its heart, neoliberal theory views individual economic liberty as the necessary basis for human wellbeing. Sovereign individuals, this theory suggests, should be unimpeded in their exercise and enjoyment of private property rights, or their capacity to trade without restriction in a free market. These normative ideas have, in turn, informed a public policy agenda associated with small states, economic deregulation, privatisation, and the active marketisation of more and more aspects of human life (Peck, 2010).

David Harvey's (2005, 64) definition of neoliberalism remains the essential point of reference:

> *a theory of political economic practices that proposes that human well-being can best be advanced by liberating individual entrepreneurial freedoms and skills within an institutional framework characterized by strong private property rights, free markets and free trade. The role of the state is to create and preserve the institutional framework appropriate to such practices ... It must ... set up those military, defence, police, and legal structures and functions required to secure private property rights and to guarantee, by force if need be, the proper functioning of markets. Furthermore, if markets do not exist (in areas such as land, water, education, health care, social security, or environmental pollution) then they must be created, by state action if necessary. But beyond these tasks the state should not venture. State interventions in markets (once created) must be kept to a bare minimum because, according to the theory, the state cannot possibly possess enough information to second-guess market signals ... and because powerful interest groups will inevitably distort and bias state interventions (particularly in democracies) for their own benefit.*

But we acknowledge that, for many, neoliberalism remains a somewhat ambiguous and contested concept, one that eludes a single, shared definition. Despite its seeming ubiquity, 'neoliberalism' can often feel like an awkward, imprecise, or excessively charged concept. And there has long been a degree of disagreement about the precise and proper meaning of the term, its conceptual clarity, and utility (Boas & Gans-Morse, 2009; Phelan, 2022; Thorsen, 2010; Venugopal, 2015). Indeed, some scholars have debated whether neoliberalism represents an analytically coherent, or conceptually distinct political theoretical tradition at all (Vallier, 2021). There would appear to be various possible reasons for this confusion and controversy.

- Firstly, neoliberalism, like many traditions of political thought, eludes clear boundaries with convergent theoretical traditions, and is internally both varied and heterogenous. In this respect, neoliberalism can be described as an "amorphous" and "loosely demarcated"

(Thorsen, 2010, 203), rather than unified, tradition; one that straddles the fault lines between classical liberalism and libertarianism and simultaneously accommodates a spectrum of related normative ideas and commitments about politics, society, and the economy.

- Secondly, 'neoliberalism' is often deployed to describe both an intellectual tradition, comprised of certain recurring normative ideas, values, and commitments, as well as a variety of real-world political projects, processes, and policy agendas discernible over recent decades (Boas & Gans-Morse, 2009; Campbell & Pederson, 2001; Gallo, 2022; Mudge, 2008; Munck, 2005; Springer, 2010). In this sense, neoliberalism can be used to refer both to theory and/or praxis; a way of conceptually identifying and categorising certain abstract ideas, and/or the ways these ideas are made real in the world through the actions and decisions of various political, social, and economic agents.

- Thirdly, neoliberalism retains a particular reputation as a concept that is perhaps deployed more for its rhetorical force than its analytical precision. Indeed, the concept of neoliberalism has been described simply as an "oppositional slogan" (Springer, 2010, 1029), and a "shorthand for everything wrong and horrible" (Thorsen, 2010, 206). As Sean Phelan notes, whilst first conceived in the 1920s, the term 'neoliberalism' only "started to gain traction—as an object of critique—in critical academic and activist circles from the 1980s onwards" (2021, 151). This association with political activism and critique remains, with very few people writing positively or sympathetically from a self-identifying 'neoliberal' position. Instead, "[p]ractically everyone who writes about neoliberalism does so as part of a critique of neoliberal ideology" (Thorsen, 2010, 189). There is therefore a sense that 'neoliberalism' may be something of a left-wing bogeyman, a general rubric for anything and everything considered wrong with contemporary capitalism and the political right, rather than a coherent tradition of political thought open to deep and sustained critical analysis.

- Finally, it could be that the conceptual contours of neoliberalism are somewhat obscured by its hegemonic ubiquity. Neoliberalism is, in this sense, "everywhere, but at the same time, nowhere" (Venugopal, 2015, 165), more difficult to analytically discern, define, and critique because neoliberal ideas, policies, and agendas have become both increasingly common place, and internalised as common sense, within our societies. This blurring of neoliberal ideas and policy agendas with popular conceptions of modernity and *realpolitik* is captured by Mark Fisher's description of "the widespread sense that not only is [neoliberal] capitalism the only viable political and economic system, but also that it is now impossible even to *imagine* a coherent alternative to it" (2009, 2 emphasis in original).

For us, much of this agonising and rumination stems from a tendency to construe neoliberalism as an object of analysis rather than a category of process. It is of course necessary to think less about neoliberalism per se and more about *neoliberalisation*. It is through grounding itself in particular milieux that neoliberalism does work in the world but in so doing its pristine philosophical purity and ideal typical institutional architecture necessarily becomes colorated, refracted, and disfigured.

In reality, there has never been a laboratory hygienic enough to live up to the billing of market fundamentalism. As Karl Polanyi insisted, markets are historically, politically, and socially constructed, always and inescapably striated and mottled and never pure, clean, and uncontaminated. Indeed, a strong state is a prerequisite for functioning liberalised markets and the market is a deeply socially engineered institution. We can speak however about the extent of market rule across capitalism's variegated histories and geographies, noting the moments when, and the places where, states have acted decisively to constitute liberalised deregulated market rule and when, in contrast, they have commanded and compensated markets. Neoliberalism signals merely the relative ascent of the former at the expense of the latter, not the wholesale replacement of the latter in favour of the former.

At the heart of the concept of 'actually existing neoliberalism' is the notion that proto-neoliberalism is an economic thought experiment which has become woven into localities in different ways as a consequence of their unique social, cultural, economic, political, and institutional histories. Neoliberalism has worked in and on fields of inherited institutional landscapes and regulatory architecture, creating situated, variegated, and uneven neoliberal penetrations and transformations. In the words of Brenner and Theodore (2002, 351), neoliberalising projects are always "produced within national, regional, and local contexts defined by the legacies of inherited institutional frameworks, policy regimes, regulatory practices and political struggles". In these divergent contexts, processes of 'creative destruction' have created new (de)regulatory environments but always in the company of, and always leveraging, inherited institutional forms.

British neoliberalism then is best understood as something of a mongrel amalgamation of emergent processes of marketisation and commoditisation (minimal state, privatisation of public services, public–private partnerships, developer/speculator led planning, low corporate and individual taxation, light to no regulation, clientelism) working in and through inherited Fordist-Keynesian institutions and social welfarism (developmental state, social partnership, welfare safety net, high taxation, regulatory obligations, planning). Its manifestations are always contextual, contingent, contested, and transient.

Holding in tension the apparent post-2008 (global financial crises) global reassertion of neoliberal hegemony and the contingent and contested production and reproduction of neoliberal regulatory instruments in particular locales, Peck, Theodore and Brenner (2013, 1093) call for work which "continues to elaborate and fine-tune an epistemological and methodological stance that is both analytically and politically disruptive, as it confronts the challenges of tracking the variegated geographies of neoliberal hegemony". In particular, they draw attention to the need to pivot attention towards place-specific manifestations of what they refer to as post-crises 'neoliberalism redux'. They note that even when aggressive market logics lead to reckless and maverick behaviours, crises, and painful fiscal adjustments, neoliberalisation has acquired a track record of finding ways to thrive and often even to flourish. Crises create in their wake new and novel neoliberal institutions forms, practices, recalibrations, and orientations—including neoliberal regulatory experiments crafted in response to shock events and the invention and institutionalisation of novel and embryonic neoliberal designs as recovery unfolds. But they note that there is nothing inevitable about disaster capitalism and neoliberalism redux; these outcomes are an active accomplishment by actors rooted in particular places and therefore unfolded unevenly. And the species of neoliberalism which is born is always new and different.

Informed by Peck and Theodore's theorisation of neoliberalism and post-crises neoliberalism redux and alert to the variegated geographies of and the importance of place-specific politico-institutional formations in post-crises regulatory experimentation and normalisation, we construe the UK's pandemic and nascent post-pandemic regulatory regime changes as comprising an ongoing series of provisional, contested, indeterminate, and contingent regulatory redesigns.

CONCLUSION

If they were not before, the limits of laissez-faire market capitalism are now becoming painfully clear. Four decades of neoliberal reform have bequeathed an economy that not only has registered at best mediocre growth rates but which has also lurched from one crisis to the next, creating endless and socially painful cycles of boom and bust. Adam Smith's historic belief that the invisible hand of the market would discipline capitalists to behave prudently and responsibly over the long term now fails to convince. A climate crisis, widening wealth and income inequalities, the rise of nationalist populist movements, and pervasive poor mental health are all symptoms of a political-economic model that is generating unsustainable negative externalities. And then has come COVID-19, a pandemic event that has been rendered more potent by dint of the UK's diminishing resilience and which in turn has further weakened the country's immune system. It is little wonder then that Simon Springer (2016, 2021) advises that it is now time to 'fuck neoliberalism...and then some'.

The multiple crises which British neoliberalism has caused or amplified, and the reciprocal damage inflicted by episodic shocks on the efficacy of the British neoliberal model, has eroded social consent for laissez-faire market capitalism and led many commentators to contemplate the possibility that we exist at a hinge point in history; a moment when the neoliberal political compact exhausts what is left of its technical and social legitimacy, and is replaced by a new social democratic regulatory regime, much in the same way as it itself replaced the failing Fordist-Keynesian compromise in the mid-1970s. Might COVID-19 prove to be the tipping point; a crisis too far?

In the early 1970s, following thirty glory years of growth in the advanced capitalist world, few would have predicted the collapse of the Fordist-Keynesian compromise. And yet it rapidly unravelled and quickly became obsolete. Like then, the system now is structurally exhausted and limping. There is no reason to think that neoliberalism will have a longer life expectancy and there is every reason to believe that we may be living at yet another fulcrum point in political-economic history. Both the technical and social performance of the neoliberal model now lacks legitimacy. Like in the 1970s, exogenous shocks are taking an already precarious system to the brink. For the OPEC oil crisis, Vietnam War, and the Iranian revolution read climate change, political populism, and now the COVID-19 pandemic. Perhaps a new social democratic project is just around the corner even if its contours are hard to imagine. The mantra 'there is no alternative' has never looked less shaky. But it would be folly to underestimate neoliberalism's staying power. Market fundamentalism has a track record of doubling down after a crisis episode and past commitments to 'build back better' have all too often morphed into disaster capitalism and neoliberalism redux.

REFERENCES

Boas, T. C., & Gans-Morse, J. (2009). Neoliberalism: From new liberal philosophy to anti-liberal slogan. *Studies in Comparative International Development, 44,* 137–161.

Brenner, N., & Theodore, N. (2002). Cities and the geographies of "Actually existing neoliberalism". *Antipode, 34*(3), 349–379.

Campbell, J. L., & Pedersen, O. K. (2001). *The rise of neoliberalism and institutional analysis.* Princeton University Press.

Esping-Andersen, G. (1990). *The three worlds of welfare capitalism.* Princeton University Press.

Fisher, M. (2009). *Capitalist realism: Is there no alternative?* Zero Books.

Gallo, E. (2022). Three varieties of authoritarian neoliberalism: Rule by the experts, the people, the leader. *Competition & Change, 26*(5), 554–574.

Hall, P. A., & Soskice, D. (Eds.). (2001). *Varieties of capitalism: The institutional foundations of comparative advantage.* OUP.

Harvey, D. (2003). *The new imperialism.* Oxford University Press.

Harvey, D. (2007). Neoliberalism as creative destruction. *The ANNALS of the American Academy of Political and Social Science, 610*(1), 21–44.

Harvey, D. (2010). *The enigma of capital and the crises of capitalism.* Oxford University Press.

Milanovic, B. (2019). Capitalism, alone: The future of the system that rules the world. Harvard University Press.

Mudge, S. L. (2008). What is neo-liberalism? *Socio-Economic Review, 6,* 703–731.

Munck, R. (2005). Neoliberalism and politics, and the politics of neoliberalism. In A. Saad-Filho & D. Johnston (Eds.), *Neoliberalism: A critical reader* (pp. 60–69). Pluto Press.

Peck, J. (2010). *Constructions of neoliberal reason.* OUP.

Peck, J. (2022). Confessions of a recovering régulation theorist. In B. Hillier, R. Philips & J. Peck (Eds.), *Regulation theory, space, and uneven development* (pp. 169–190). 1984Press.

Peck, J., & Theodore, N. (2019). Still neoliberalism? *South Atlantic Quarterly, 118*(2), 245–265.

Peck, J., Theodore, N., & Brenner, N. (2013). Neoliberal urbanism redux? *International Journal of Urban and Regional Research, 37*(3), 1091–1099.

Phelan, S. (2022). What's in a name? Political antagonism and critiquing 'neoliberalism', *Journal of Political Ideologies, 27*(2), 148–167.

Piore, M., & Sabel, C. F. (1984). *The second industrial divide: Possibilities for prosperity*. Basic Books.

Springer, S. (2010). Neoliberalism and geography: Expansions, variegations, formations. *Geography Compass, 4*(8), 1025–1038.

Springer, S. (2016). Fuck neoliberalism. *ACME: An International Journal for Critical Geographies, 15*(2), 285–292.

Springer, S. (2021). *Fuck neoliberalism: Translating resistance*. PM Press.

Taylor, F. W. (1911). *The principles of scientific management*. Harper & Brothers.

Thorsen, D. E. (2010). The neoliberal challenge: What is neoliberalism? *Contemporary Readings in Law and Social Justice, 2*(2), 188–214.

Vallier, K. (2021). Neoliberalism. https://plato.stanford.edu/archives/sum 2021/entries/neoliberalism/. Accessed 28 Dec 2021.

Venugopal, R. (2015). Neoliberalism as concept. *Economy and Society, 44*(2), 165–187.

CHAPTER 3

Chastened: The UK's Encounter with COVID-19 in Global Context

Abstract In this chapter we draw upon data on confirmed COVID-19 cases, deaths, and excess deaths to map and interrogate the global and still emergent spatio-temporal trajectories of the COVID-19 pandemic. We document in particular the travails of advanced liberal market democracies relative to the rest of the world and the travails of the UK relative to other advanced liberal market democracies. Our investigation points to a complex picture that defies cursory summary. Nonetheless, with noteable exceptions and important qualifications and caveats, there is more than sufficient evidence we submit, to support the hypothesis that COVID-19 has exacted an unexpectedly heavy toll on more developed Global North high-income advanced liberal market democracies and that neoliberal states including the UK have been particularly impacted.

Keywords COVID-19's global geographies · COVID-19 deaths · COVID-19 excess deaths · OECD · United Kingdom · Data

INTRODUCTION

On December 31, 2019, the Wuhan Municipal Health Commission reported to the World Health Organisation (WHO) the existence of a cluster of pneumonia cases in Wuhan, Hubei Province, China. Shortly

M. Boyle et al., *COVID-19 and the Case Against Neoliberalism*, https://doi.org/10.1007/978-3-031-18935-7_3

43

thereafter severe acute respiratory syndrome coronavirus 2 or SARS-CoV-2 was identified as the responsible pathogen and the disease itself was given the label COVID-19. An epidemiological event of world historical importance was to begin.

By January 30, 2020, WHO reported a total of 7818 confirmed cases across 18 countries (but almost all in China) and 43 confirmed deaths (again, almost all in China). That same day, WHO declared COVID-19 a Public Health Emergency of International Concern (PHEIC). By March 11, 2020, 118,000 confirmed cases had been recorded in 110 countries, resulting in over 19,000 confirmed deaths. On that day, WHO upgraded COVID-19 to the status of a global pandemic. Alas it has since lived up to its billing. By June 30, 2020, 10.5 million confirmed cases and 536,512 confirmed deaths had been recorded; by June 30, 2021, this had risen to 182.3 million cases and 3.95 million deaths, and by June 30, 2022, 548.2 million cases and 6.35 million deaths.

This chapter places under scrutiny the spatio-temporal diffusion of COVID-19 from its initial epicentre in Wuhan. Whilst the pandemic has been global in its reach, it has undoubtedly crashed onto some shores with greater ferocity and fecundity than others and a number of patterns are starting to become manifest. We will see that COVID-19 has exacted an unexpectedly heavy toll on more developed Global North high-income advanced liberal market democracies and that neoliberal states including the UK have been particularly impacted. But tellingly, not all advanced liberal market democracies and not all neoliberalising states performed poorly and poor outcomes were not limited to states wedded to market fundamentalism. Moreover, the performance of the advanced capitalist world including and in particular the UK, has varied over time: outcomes have progressively improved, albeit in a non-linear way. And many of these countries have avoided large scale secondary or 'downstream' excess deaths.

We once again, then, underscore the central thesis advanced in this book: whilst insisting on the need to situate government responses to COVID-19 in the context of the logics and legacies of forty years of neoliberal rule, it is equally important to recognise that these responses are always contingent and active accomplishments. Political philosophies provide historical actors with choice architectures but it is political leaders who in the end make choices. Path dependency does not equal path lock-in—things could have been, and may yet be, different.

Mapping COVID-19's Global Geographies: In Search of a Method

When mapping COVID-19's evolving geographies, we have been forced to make a number of methodological choices; these choices require explicit registering from the outset as they set limits on the claims that we are able to make in this chapter.

To understand fully the damage inflicted by the global pandemic on different places, it would be necessary to attend not only to its immediate public health impacts but also to its cascading political, economic, social, cultural, technological, and environmental aftershocks. This task, however, extends beyond the scope of this study. We will note of course that health and non-health impacts are deeply inter-related; the former has precipitated the latter and the latter has mediated the former. But our focus will be confined strictly to the public health crisis and its remediation. Our central objective is to map and interpret the variegated impacts of COVID-19 on rates of morbidity and mortality among national populations.

Global comparative analysis of COVID-19 health outcomes is severely hampered by data limitations. The World Health Organization (WHO), Johns Hopkins Coronavirus Resource Centre (CRC), the US Centre for Disease Control (CDC), and the European Centre for Disease Prevention and Control (ECDC) provide the most authoritative, up-to-date data on COVID-19 cases and deaths at the global scale. The Human Mortality Database's Short-term Mortality Fluctuations (STMF) data series (co-produced by UC Berkeley and the Max Planck Institute in Germany) and the World Mortality Dataset (produced by Ariel Karlinsky and Dmitry Kobak) provide data on excess deaths but cover only 38 countries and 120 countries, respectively, and exclude many important African and Asian countries. More 'global' sets of *estimates* of excess deaths are produced by the Economist (187 countries), the Institute of Health Metrics and Evaluation) (IHME) (191 countries), and the WHO (194 countries).

In each and every case, national data sets are pooled. Because the quantity and quality of health data varies from country to country, this pooled data lacks common standards, inter-operability, and by implication authority. In response, and in advance of the next global pandemic, the World Health Organisation has established a new Hub for Pandemic and Epidemic Intelligence, based in Berlin. For now, however, we must work with the data we have got.

Our objective is to place the liberal democratic advanced capitalist world in global context and the UK in the context of the liberal democratic advanced capitalist world. As such, we are particularly concerned that given their stronger institutional capacities and democratic obligations, highly developed Global North countries may be more likely to test, register, and report COVID-19 cases and deaths than their less developed Global South counterparts. Mapping COVID-19's global diffusion using national data sets runs the risk of over-emphasising the scale of the pandemic in high-income advanced democratic economies and under-estimating the burden of COVID-19 on the health of people living in lower income countries and especially low-income autocracies. Substantive conclusions might be drawn in error; apparent trends may arise simply as an artefact of geographical variations in data capacities and practices.

Is this concern warranted? With respect to the Global South, there are concerns that data published by some African, Asian, and to a lesser extent Latin American governments look awry; when reporting COVID-19 outcomes, some national census offices face not only technical but also political challenges. But many Global South countries have excellent epidemiological data infrastructures and so we must not fall prey to casual and prejudicial assumptions about the quality of data generated beyond the advanced capitalist world. Meanwhile, such is the novelty of COVID-19 that data collection has undoubtedly been more haphazard even across the Global North than would normally be the case and national data are likely to be incomplete and subject to future re-correction. There is no reason to assume that data collected in other advanced market democracies is especially inferior or misleading when compared to data collected in the UK. Comparative analysis *within* the Global North can surely be undertaken with a reasonable amount of confidence that the data is indeed manifesting meaningful insights.

Can we mitigate this concern? Whilst we examine trends in each of the recorded cases, deaths, and excess deaths in the UK, when undertaking international comparative analysis, we place more emphasis on the latter two, death rates and excess death rates. We judge recorded cases to be measured so variably by countries as to render comparison futile. Of course, death rates are likely to be subject to severe limitations too. According to WHO, the percentage of registered deaths ranges from 98% in some EU countries to only 10% in some countries in Africa. But death certification is more universally practised and standardised (at present, still to the WHO's International Classification of Diseases 10th Revision).

More concerning is the fact that definitions of what constitutes a COVID-19 death vary from country to country. In the UK, for instance, official data reports deaths that occur within 28 days of a positive test, although some data sets include deaths that occur within 60 days of a positive result whilst others again include only deaths where COVID-19 is referenced in the death certification. But we would argue that statistics on mortality are likely to yield more purposeful conclusions than those on cases. Meanwhile, whilst estimates of excess deaths (defined as the difference between the observed numbers of deaths in specific time periods and expected numbers of deaths (on the basis of historical trends) vary between studies and are open to interpretation, there is no doubt that this measure offers a potentially powerful antidote to uneven geographies of data quantity and quality.

By self-admission, our investigation suffers from a degree of methodological nationalism and glosses over important subnational variations in processes, responses, and outcomes. This limitation bears on this study in especially acute ways. We recognise that, as a result of their devolved policy responsibilities, there have been significant variations in the way governments in England, Scotland, Wales, and Northern Ireland have responded to the pandemic. Nevertheless, for the sake of parsimony, in this paper we focus our analysis on the national (UK) government and its response to COVID-19. Where, because of devolution, the UK government's policies and decisions during the pandemic have taken effect in England only, we have tried to make this clear. We have also included analysis of subnational data sets in Chapter 7 where we discuss regional inequalities in wealth, income, and COVID-19 outcomes.

To locate the performance of the advanced capitalist world in global context and the performance of the UK with respect to other advanced capitalist liberal democracies, we refer in our commentary to the OECD grouping in particular; an institution promoting best practice in Western economic policy and perhaps the most appropriate proxy of the geographical limits of the imagined community of the West (Map 3.1). But our coverage goes much wider. We undertake analysis on the basis of a range of Western leaning territorial units or blocs. Each bloc embodies one or more institutional pillars commonly associated with liberal market democracy; because they vary in mission and composition, they each nevertheless tell us something distinctive about why high-income Global North countries have presented as surprisingly vulnerable. Using the themes of health; economy, development, and income; democracy, liberalism, and

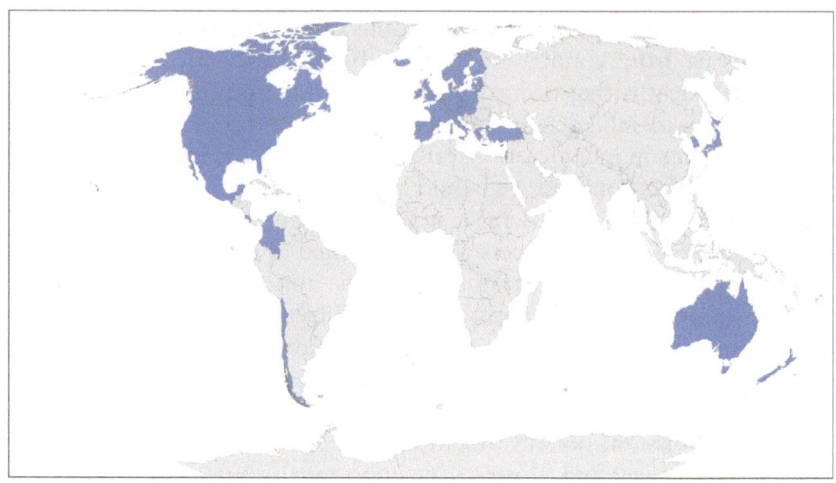

Map 3.1 Map of OECD member countries (*Source* Authors' own)

freedom; power, influence, and leadership; and imperialism, history, and culture, we examine trends in COVID-19 deaths and excess deaths for each of the WHO's European Region, the World Bank High Income grouping, high ranking countries in the United Nations Human Development Index (HDI), International Monetary Fund (IMF) Advanced Economies, the Organisation for Economic Cooperation and Development (OECD) world, high ranking countries in each of the V-Dem political regimes (liberal democracy) classification, the Cato/Frazer Human Freedom Index, the DHL Global Connectivity Index, the Economist Democracy Index, the North Atlantic Treaty Organisation (NATO) bloc, EU27, G20, G7, Paris Club, Portland30, and other large Anglophone countries (see Table 3.1 and Appendix for further details).

When examining trends in the impact of the pandemic on public health in national population stocks around the world, we have come to realise that interpretation is sensitive to the slice of time we chose to place under scrutiny. Conclusions reached by confining analysis to only one time period can, in fact, paint a misleading picture; the full landscape might only come to the fore by adopting narrower and/or wider temporal frames. Having run multiple analyses over multiple and overlapping time periods, we believe the time windows we make use of in our analysis below

Table 3.1 Guide to geographical units/territorial blocs referred to in this chapter

Theme	Geographical units of analysis and associated data sets
Global base data	UN Member States $n = 193$ Total population = 7.85 billion The United Kingdom (UK) Total population 0.068 billion
Health	WHO European Region countries $n = 53$ Total population 0.89 billion
Economy, Development, Income	World Bank High Income countries $n = 80$ Total population = 1.27 billion
	United Nations Human Development Index $n = 30$ (top ranked countries) Total population = 0.89 billion
	International Monetary Fund (IMF) Advanced Economies $n = 40$ Total population 1.1 billion
	The Organisation for Economic Co-operation and Development (OECD) Advanced Liberal Market Democracies $n = 38$ Total population 1.36 billion
Democracy, Liberalism, Freedom	V-Dem Institute Liberal Democracy Index (LDI) and Regimes of Democracy $n = 34$ Total population 1.3 billion
	Cato Institute/Fraser Institute Human Freedom Index 2021 $n = 30$ Total population 0.95 billion
	DHL Global Connectivity Index $n = 30$ Total population 1.32 billion
Power, Influence, Leadership	North Atlantic Treaty Organisation (NATO) $n = 30$ Total population 0.94 billion
	European Union EU27 $n = 27$ Total population 0.45 billion
	G20 World's Largest Advanced and Emerging Economies $n = 19 +$ EU Total population 4.7 billion
	G7 Major Advanced Economies $n = 7$ Total Population 700 million
	The Paris Club $n = 22$ Total population 1.32 billion
Imperialism, History, Culture	Large Anglophone countries $n = 7$ Total population 0.55 billion

Source Authors' own

afford a fair and balanced insight into global trends in COVID-19, especially as they bear on the UK. Dates readers might care to take note of are:

- *January 1, 2020 to June 30, 2022 The time period over which analysis has been undertaken for this book.*
- *January 29, 2020 Date of the first confirmed COVID-19 case in the UK.*
- *February 18, 2020 Date of the first confirmed COVID-19 death in the OECD and EU (Italy).*
- *March 5, 2020 The first COVID-19 death recorded in the UK.*
- *March 11, 2020 Date when COVID-19 was designated by the WHO as a 'global pandemic'.*
- *January 31, 2020 to July 31, 2020 The UK's first wave, covering a 6 month period from the country's first recorded case.*
- *March 23, 2020 to July 19, 2021 The period from the first national lockdown to 'Freedom Day' when restrictions were lifted (initially in England), including the UK's first and second waves.*
- *July 19, 2021 to June 30, 2022 The period from 'Freedom Day' to the date of completion of this book which includes the UK's fourth wave (Omicron), introduction of lighter 'Plan B' restrictions, and gradual easing back to pre-pandemic normality.*
- *Dominant variants in the UK. January 2020 to December 2020 Multiple, January 2021 to May 2021 Alpha, May 2021 to December 2021 Delta, and December 2022 to June 2022 Omicron.*
- *December 8, 2020 First person in the UK gets (Pfizer) vaccine. June 30, 2021 50% of the UK population fully vaccinated. June 30, 2022 75% of the UK population fully vaccinated.*

Finally, we emphasise once again that acute problems attend to the analysis of what is a dynamic and rapidly evolving situation. Only when the pandemic has been permanently suppressed will we be in a position to reflect upon its final patterns of diffusion across time and over space.

The UK's Encounter with COVID-19: Key Trends in Cases and Deaths

The first case of COVID-19 in the UK was confirmed on January 31, 2020, and the first death on March 5, 2020. Figure 3.1 documents subsequent COVID-19 cases and deaths, vaccination rates, and patients in ICU, across what might be described as four distinctive pandemic waves and associated spikes and troughs.

The first wave began in earnest in early March 2020. Confirmed cases peaked on April 26, 2020, at 4846 per day, whilst confirmed deaths peaked at 983 per day on April 15. By June, the UK government had flattened the curve with confirmed cases falling to 356 per day by July 6, 2020, whilst confirmed deaths troughed at 7 per day 6 weeks later, on August 21st. At the end of the first wave, a cumulative total of 322,884 cases and 41,453 deaths had been recorded.

Notwithstanding this progress, from July 31 and especially from August 31, 2020, confirmed cases began to rise again, and from September 5, 2020, so too confirmed deaths. This second wave appeared to have peaked on November 10, 2020, at 22,785 confirmed cases per day and on November 28 at 486 confirmed deaths per day. By December 3, 2020, confirmed cases had fallen to 14,237 per day and by December 15 confirmed deaths troughed at 411 per day. Respite was to be short-lived. As winter took hold and especially across the 2020/2021 Christmas break, this second wave itself developed a second wind which proved to be more severe than the initial surge. A sharp rise in confirmed cases led to peaks of 59,809 per day on January 10th and confirmed deaths reached a pinnacle of 1263 on January 24, 2021. From these heights, the pandemic began to be brought under control, greatly accelerated by a rapidly deployed vaccine programme. Lows of 1850 confirmed cases and 6 confirmed deaths per day were recorded on May 20, 2021, and May 23, 2021, respectively. As the second wave petered out, a cumulative total of 322,884 cases and 41,453 deaths had been recorded.

From July 1, 2021, a third wave emerged which followed a distinctively new trajectory. Across the period to December 1, 2021, new confirmed cases and deaths slowly grew in number but instead of peaking they oscillated at a sustained high of 35,000–45,000 per day and 100–165 per day, respectively. By the end of this third wave, a cumulative of 10.35 million confirmed cases and 145,385 confirmed deaths had been registered.

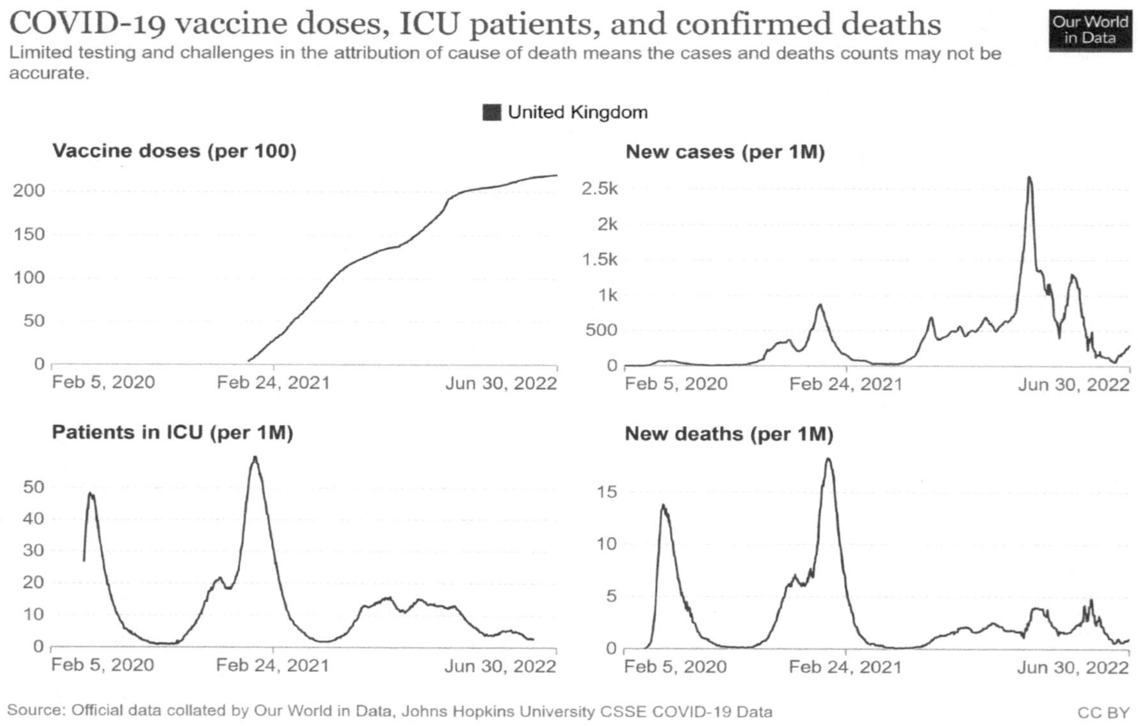

COVID-19 vaccine doses, ICU patients, and confirmed deaths

Limited testing and challenges in the attribution of cause of death means the cases and deaths counts may not be accurate.

■ United Kingdom

Vaccine doses (per 100)

New cases (per 1M)

Patients in ICU (per 1M)

New deaths (per 1M)

Source: Official data collated by Our World in Data, Johns Hopkins University CSSE COVID-19 Data   CC BY

Fig. 3.1 Confirmed COVID-19 cases, deaths, ICU patients and vaccine doses in the UK, 7-day rolling averages, January 2020–June 2022 (*Source* John Hopkins University CSSE COVID-19 Data)

This wave was not to fall away and trough however and with the arrival of the Omicron variant a step change in confirmed cases and deaths per day were to further escalate what was an already alarming and stubborn high. Between December 2021 and April 2022—punctured by a limited lockdown-related valley between mid-January and mid-March 2022—confirmed cases rapidly rose to the twin peaks at 181,687 per day (January 6, 2022) and 88,984 per day (March 21, 2022) and confirmed deaths to 266 per day (January 19, 2022) and 328 per day (April 25, 2022). The fourth wave now looks to have receded and on June 30, 2022, confirmed cases and deaths per day have fallen to 21,566 and 66, respectively. On this day, a cumulative total of 22.82 million confirmed cases and 180,424 confirmed deaths had been recorded.

Although varying in extent, the UK's four nations broadly followed the four wave sequence described (Fig. 3.2). Wales would appear to have repeatedly topped the peaks of the four waves and endured (by June 2022) the highest confirmed cumulative deaths at 338 per 100,000. By comparison, Northern Ireland managed to flatten the curve and restrict cases and deaths particularly successfully in waves 1 and 2 and witnessed confirmed cumulative death rates of 250 per 100,000. For most of the pandemic Scotland better than England and Wales but hit a higher peak in wave 4, resulting in a confirmed cumulative death rate of 281 per 100,000. Finally, England performed comparatively poorly in waves 1 and 2 but comparatively better in waves 3 and 4 (from June 2021 onwards death rates were generally lower in England than in Scotland, Wales, and Northern Ireland); the result was a cumulative confirmed rate of 297.25 per 100,000 on June 30, 2022.

The relationship between cases, deaths, hospitalisations, and ICU admissions has clearly varied across the four waves.

The UK government struggled to subdue the pandemic during its first and second waves and too many COVID-19 cases were translated into COVID-19 deaths across 2020 in particular. The rollout of a vaccine from early 2021 appears to have had little impact on confirmed cases which peaked at their highest levels during the fourth wave. The UK government however evidently gained a capacity over time to break the link between cases and deaths, and case fatality rates have declined systematically over time. At the peak of the first wave confirmed cases per day were relatively low but confirmed deaths were exceptionally high (case fatality rates of 14%); confirmed cases were comparatively higher in the second

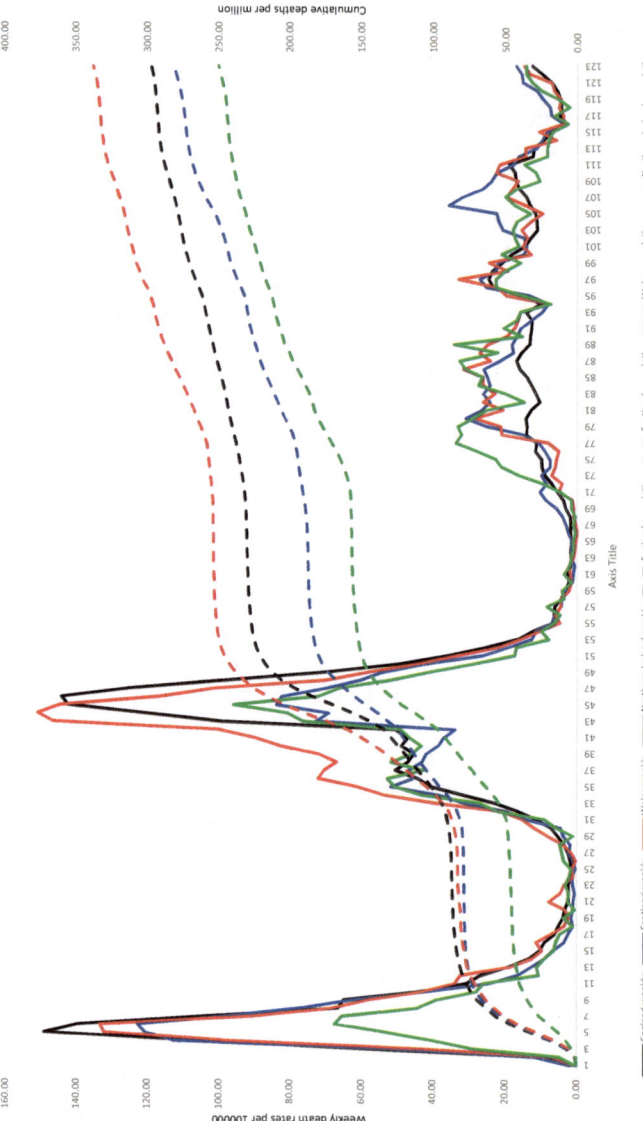

Fig. 3.2 Weekly death rates per 100000 and cumulative death rates per million across the UK by nation March 2020 to June 2022

wave but confirmed deaths again were very high (case fatality rates of circa 3.5% at peak); by the third wave both confirmed cases and deaths peaked at lower levels and became more aligned (case fatality rate of 1.5% at peak), and finally during wave four confirmed cases exploded to an all-time high but confirmed deaths declined to an all-time low (case fatality rates less than 1%).

The vaccine programme and enhanced therapeutics appear to have had a transformative impact on serious illness (subduing hospitalisations, ICU admissions, and deaths) especially in wave four. But the severing of the link between cases and deaths also coincides with the rise of the less virulent omicron variant. It is difficult to distinguish the relative significance of each causal variable. But it is worth noting that the vaccine rollout programme was less successful in suppressing the translation of cases into deaths in wave three when the delta variant dominated.

In part because of this observation, the capacity of the UK to continue to reduce case numbers overall and sever links between cases and deaths is not a given. The process is not linear and whilst there is cause for hope and optimism, the pandemic is far from over. Should there be an improvement in the efficacy of vaccines and/or improved therapeutics and/or if there emerges a new and less transmissible/less virulent variant—case numbers and case fatality rates may themselves drop to new lows and the UK could be facing very low levels of death and a transition to a post-pandemic period in which the country learns to live with COVID-19. Should there be a decline in the efficacy of vaccines and/or if there emerges a new and more transmissible/more virulent mutant variant—even allowing for improved therapeutics—with cases surging to new highs (July 2022), it is possible that worse may be yet to come, and that the UK potentially remains at risk of high levels of death and unsustainably high case fatality rates.

Mapping COVID-19's Uneven Global Health Impact Geographies

Global Geographies of Confirmed COVID-19 Deaths

Our approach compares actual COVID-19 death rates by country—and on the basis of a variety of Western minded territorial blocs—with the death rates which might be expected in each case had COVID-19 diffused

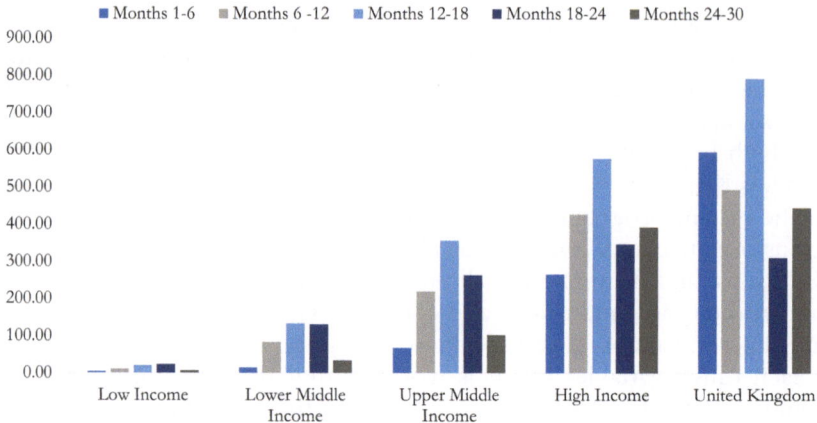

Fig. 3.3 Confirmed COVID-19 deaths per million in six month intervals January 2020–June 2022. The United Kingdom in the context of World Bank Income Regions (*Source* John Hopkins University CSSE COVID-19 Data)

evenly over the surface of the earth, varying only in proportion to population size. We assume countries and blocs reporting actual COVID-19 death rates that (far) exceed expected death rates to be COVID-19 hot spots (disproportionately burdened by the pandemic). In contrast, countries and blocs reporting COVID-19 death rates that fall (well) below that which they might expect given their population size might be understood to be COVID-19 hinterlands (escaping with lighter-than-average disease burdens).

On this basis and to the extent that data on COVID-19 deaths per capita by country/bloc are reliable enough to be instructive, we might conclude—with a degree of disbelief—that COVID-19 does indeed appear to have been more of a communicable disease of the highly developed Global North than one of the lesser developed Global South and that within the Global North the UK has presided over particularly poor outcomes (Figs. 3.3, 3.4 and Maps 3.2, 3.3, see also Appendix).

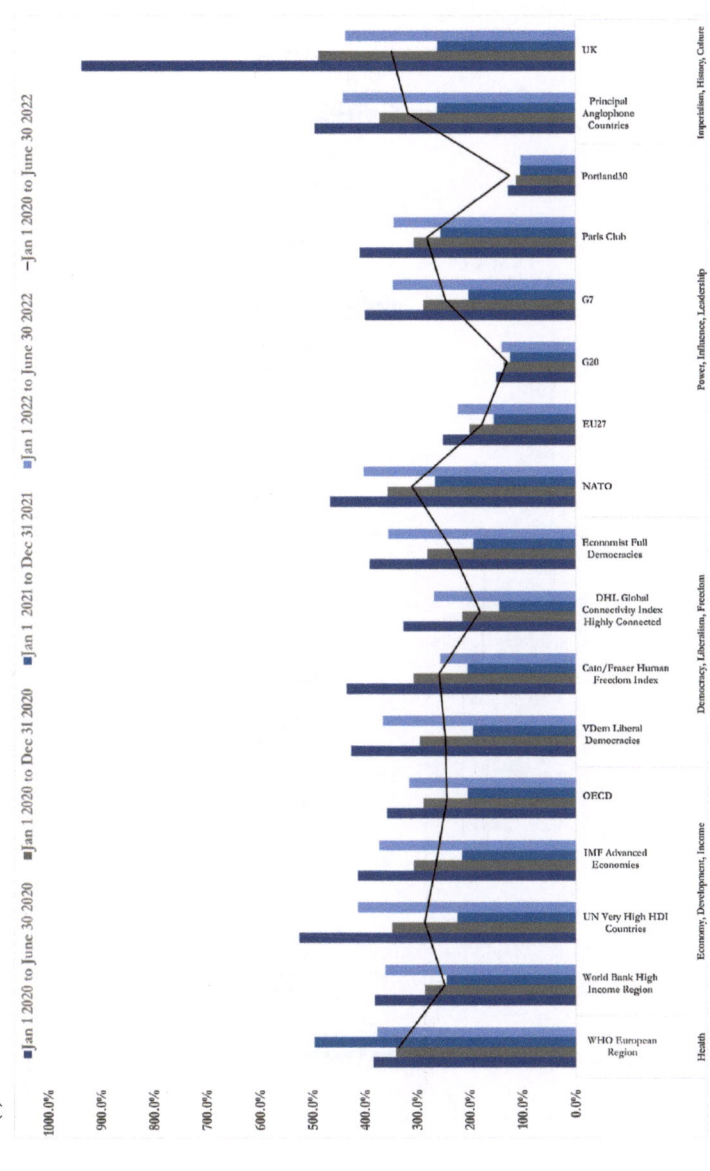

Fig. 3.4 Ratio (in %) of actual % share of confirmed COVID-19 deaths relative to % share of COVID-19 deaths which would have occurred had COVID-19 spread evenly varying only by population size. **a** Territorial blocs in global context (assumes global death toll to be distributed by population size) January 2020–June 2022. **b** UK in the context of various globally significant Western territorial units/blocs (assumes death tolls in each bloc is spread across the bloc evenly according to population size) January 2020–June 2022

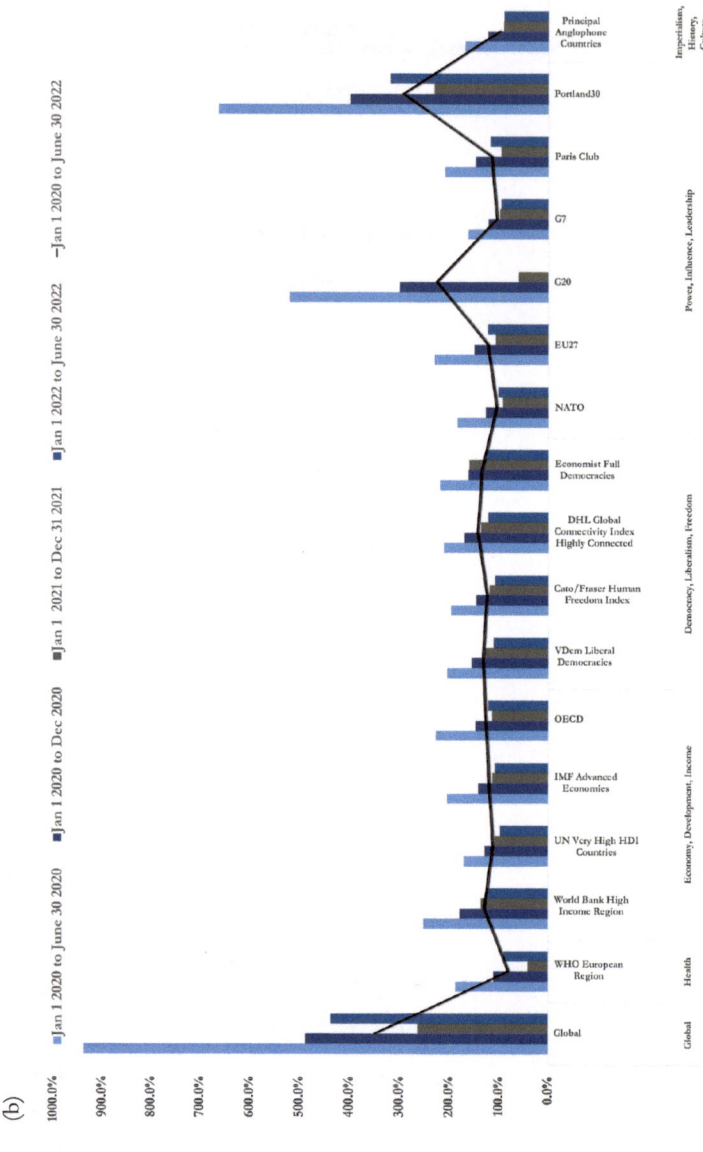

(b)

Fig. 3.4 (continued)

Cumulative confirmed COVID-19 cases per million people, Jun 30, 2022
Due to limited testing, the number of confirmed cases is lower than the true number of infections.

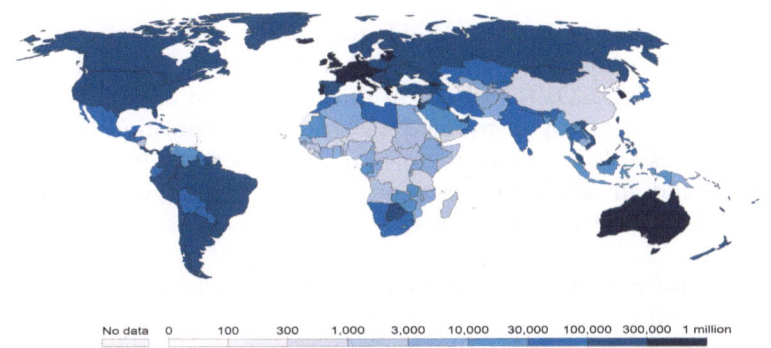

No data   0   100   300   1,000   3,000   10,000   30,000   100,000 300,000 1 million

Map 3.2   Cumulative confirmed COVID-19 cases per million people, June 30, 2022 (*Source* Johns Hopkins University CSSE COVID-19 Data)

Cumulative confirmed COVID-19 deaths per million people, Jun 30, 2022
Due to varying protocols and challenges in the attribution of the cause of death, the number of confirmed deaths may not accurately represent the true number of deaths caused by COVID-19.

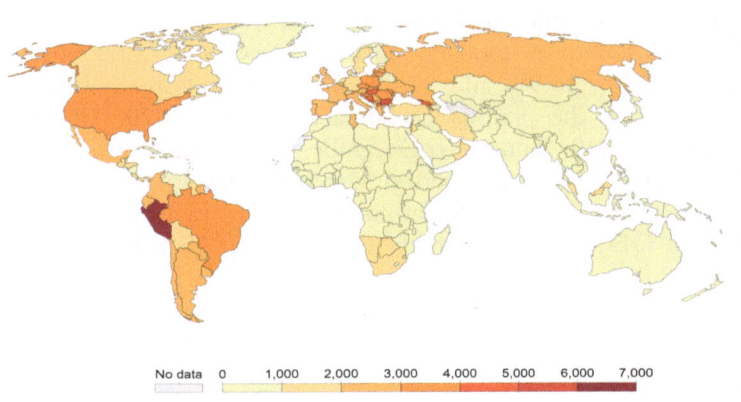

No data   0   1,000   2,000   3,000   4,000   5,000   6,000   7,000

Map 3.3   Cumulative confirmed COVID-19 deaths per million people, June 30, 2022 (*Source* Johns Hopkins University CSSE COVID-19 Data)

Advanced liberal market democracies in global context

- Across the first year of the pandemic (2020), most of the Western leaning territorial blocs we examined endured between 3 and 5 times the confirmed COVID-19 deaths they might have expected had the disease been evenly distributed according to population size; over 2021 these blocs continued to bear 2 and 3 times their expected share and in 2022 (to June 30) they presided over confirmed COVID-19 death rates between 3 and 4.5 times their expected share.
- Across the period January 2020–June 2022, the discrepancy between actual and expected confirmed COVID-19 death rates was consistently higher across the WHO's European Region (which includes Russia, Eastern Europe, and Central Asia) and the Anglophone world (which includes the US, UK, and South Africa). In the power, influence, and leadership blocs, whilst still witnessing above global average per capita death rates, the EU27 (relatively more social democratic in orientation), and G20, and Portland30 blocs (which include a broader range of powerful non-Western global actors) appear to have achieved better outcomes.
- With only 18% of the global population, the OECD world registered 64.6%, 52.0%, 36.9%, and 57.0% of global confirmed COVID-19 deaths across the periods of January to June 2020, January to December 2020, January to December 2021, and January to June 2022, respectively. In the period March 5, 2020 to March 5, 2021, the top ten countries (population >1 million) by deaths per capita were all OECD countries and 18 of the top 25 belonged to the OECD.

The UK in the context of the advanced liberal market democracies

- During the first six months of the pandemic (January to June 2020), with only 0.8% of the global population, the UK registered 7.5% of all confirmed COVID-19 deaths, nearly ten times the deaths it might have expected had COVID-19 been distributed evenly over space on a per capita basis. Across the whole of 2020, this figure was nearly

5 times, across 2021 over 2.5 times, and in the first six months of 2022 over 4 times.

- When set into the context of the advanced capitalist world it is evident that the UK also ranks amongst the West's poorest performers. With the exception of the WHO's European Region (which includes Russia and Central Asian and Eastern European countries) and the Anglophone bloc (which includes the US and South Africa), the UK has consistently recorded more deaths per capita than the average for a wide range of Western blocs. In the power, influence, and leadership bloc, whilst still witnessing above global average per capita death rates, the EU27 (relatively more social democratic in orientation) and the G20 and Portland30 blocs (again which incorporates non-Western global powers) appear to have achieved better outcomes.
- With only 5.1% of the OECD population, in the first six months of the pandemic (to June 2020) the UK recorded 11.6% of all its COVID-19 deaths and across all of 2020 registered 7.5% of all deaths. Across the entire period January 2020 to June 2022, the UK recorded 127.3% of the deaths it might have expected if had achieved outcomes on a par with the OECD average. On June 30, 2020, December 31, 2020, June 30, 2021, December 31, 2021, and June 30, 2022, respectively, amongst OECD member states the UK was ranked 3/38, 5/38, 8/38, 12/38, and 13/38 for COVID-19 deaths per capita.

So, what—if anything—might global geographies of confirmed COVID-19 death rates tell us about the extent of the burden of disease shouldered by Western liberal market democracies generally and the UK specifically?

In terms of confirmed deaths per capita, COVID-19 has indeed weighed disproportionately upon the liberal market democracies of the Global North, and the UK has indeed been amongst their worst performers. Uneven geographies of confirmed COVID-19 deaths have been to an extent levelling up over time, but they still persist. Across 2020 there can be no doubt that, notwithstanding its comparative strengths, with respect to confirmed COVID-19 deaths the UK was one of the most dangerous places on earth to live. By rolling out a vaccine campaign earlier than virtually every other country—developed and under-developed alike—the UK has gradually reduced its disproportionately large share of the global burden of disease. But still, across the full period January 2020 to June 2022, it recorded death rates that were well above the global average and the average for a wide range of Western-leaning Global North blocs.

But immediately, it is necessary to qualify and temper this conclusion by attending to variations in the prevalence and lethality of COVID-19 across capitalism's geographies. By and large, corporatist statist (European) and social democratic (Nordic) capitalisms have weathered the storm better than liberal laissez-faire market (liberal meritocratic) capitalisms. Whilst many liberalised market economies have witnessed relatively poor outcomes (US, UK, Chile), some have enjoyed comparatively better results (Australia, Ireland, and Canada). Equally, whilst many coordinated market economies have performed relatively poorly (France, Belgium, Spain), others have achieved better outcomes (for example, Japan, Taiwan South Korea, and to an extent Germany and the Netherlands). Moreover, whilst the social democratic Nordic countries of Norway, Denmark, and Finland (and here we place too New Zealand) have performed well, Sweden has trodden a different path and presided over poorer outcomes.

Beyond the advanced capitalist economies, the virus has exacted a very heavy toll in other less mature capitalist countries and emerging democracies.

Latin America—historically the most developed region within the Global South—has been particularly impacted, especially Peru, Brazil, Mexico, Colombia, Chile, Argentina, Panama, and Bolivia. Of course, of all the continents, Latin America has been most impacted by the Washington Consensus development agenda, and from the mid-1970s has been on the receiving end of a suite of fiscally conservative Structural Adjustment Programmes (SAPs). In consequence, this continent's complex admixture of hybrid capitalisms has deposited in its wake some of the sharpest wealth and income inequalities in the world. Meanwhile, for most of 2020, the transitioning hybrid market economies of Eastern Europe appeared to have had escaped the worst of the pandemic. But more recently they have witnessed extraordinary waves and peaks and are now amongst the most adversely affected (especially Bulgaria, Georgia, Hungary, Poland, Czechia Slovenia, Slovakia, North Macedonia, Romania). Why these fledging and embryonic market democracies witnessed a deferred escalation in confirmed COVID-19 death rates and why they now sit atop the global league is not altogether clear. But certainly, there would appear to be scope for these countries to further build the capacity of their still nascent transition(ing) institutions.

And what of countries aligned to alternative political, cultural, and economic systems?

By and large, 'emerging' Asia has coped better with the pandemic than other continents. Many East and Southeast Asian states have proven capable of mounting fast and effective responses to the pandemic (including Vietnam, China, Japan, South Korea, and Taiwan). Given that the countries straddling this region encompass a wide range of politico-economic-institutional models, the inference may be that specifically 'Asian' cultural factors (perhaps with respect to communal obligations, reverence towards the elderly, and respect for authority) are at work. But Malaysia appears to be a notable exception. Elsewhere in Asia, India, Pakistan, Myanmar, and Indonesia have encountered much lighter COVID-19 burdens than Russia, Iran, Georgia, and Kazakhstan. African exceptionalism is perhaps the most surprising feature of COVID-19's geographies. To the extent that the data is meaningful enough to allow us to draw conclusions, it comes as a welcome surprise that, against all odds, it is the countries which hitherto have been perceived to be especially vulnerable to communicable disease—Sub-Saharan African countries (including the very poor and very populous countries of the Democratic Republic of Congo, Malawi, and Nigeria)—which at least to this point have escaped the worst of the pandemic. Interestingly, it is countries in Africa which most proximate with liberal market democracies that have been most adversely impacted, especially South Africa, Botswana, Namibia, Tunisia and to a lesser extent Ghana and Côte d'Ivoire.

Reading across continents, some commentators have drawn attention to the role of autocratic rule, political populism, and age dependency ratios as progenitors of COVID-19 geographies. The status of these potential causal factors however is not easily established.

- Given their greater capacity and latitude to swiftly impose highly stringent and effective lockdowns amongst their populations, it has become popular to assert that authoritarian governance models lie behind the comparative success of states such as China and Vietnam in suppressing the virus. But equally, the Russian model of command capitalism and the autocratic patriarchal monarchies and theocracies which prevail in the Arabian Peninsula and the Middle East (Saudi

Arabia, Qatar, Oman, Iran, and Yemen) have been less successful in controlling the pandemic.

- Might the rise of political populism and populist governments—alleged by some to be less competent—diminished the efficacy of some countries' COVID-19 responses? Again, the picture is complex; whilst the UK, US, Hungary, Poland, and Brazil have witnessed very poor outcomes, India and the Philippines have achieved much better outcomes. Moreover, when set into their regional contexts (Eastern Europe, South America, Central, and South-East Asia), Hungary, Poland, Brazil, India, and the Philippines' COVID-19 death rates do not look that distinctive or out of place.

- And finally, what about the importance of age structure and age-related underlying conditions? Here we simply note that with a median age of 40.8 years, the UK has presided over poorer public health outcomes than Japan (median age 48.2), Germany (46.6), Hong Kong (44.8), South Korea (43.6), the Netherlands (43.2), Finland (42.8), Singapore (42.4), Denmark (42.3), Taiwan (42.2), Canada (41.3), and Norway (39.6) and outcomes similar to Italy (47.9), Portugal (46.2), Greece (45.3), France (42.0), Poland and Belgium (each 41.8). Meanwhile, countries with similar youthful age profiles appear to have presided over significantly different outcomes; whilst the Latin American countries of Peru (median age 29.1), Brazil (33.5), Argentina (31.9), and Mexico (29.3) all shouldered a disproportionately higher burden of disease, the Middle East/Arab world countries witnessed a mixed performance with Iran (32.4), Israel (30.6), and Libya (29.0) burdened much more significantly than Saudi Arabia (31.9), Qatar (31.9), and Algeria (29.1). Meanwhile, the Asian countries of Vietnam (32.6), India (28.2), Indonesia (29.3), Myanmar (29.1), and Laos (24.4) all achieved confirmed COVID-19 death rates well below the global average. But public health outcomes were comparatively more severe in Malaysia (29.1), and with an average age of 40.1, Thailand endured only 40% of the death rates recorded in Malaysia.

Global Geography of Excess Deaths

According to some epidemiologists and health statisticians, given variegated testing, recording, and reporting regimes, the only truly meaningful indicator of the impact of COVID-19 on human health is that of 'excess deaths'. Again, excess deaths can be defined as the difference between the observed numbers of deaths recorded in a specific time period and the number of deaths which might be expected in the same time period based on historical trends. But computing the scale of excess deaths is itself a problematic endeavour and different methods and measures have the potential to convey different messages.

The IHME and WHO have computed excess deaths for 2020 and 2021, whilst the Economist provides estimates for the full period January 2020 to June 2022. Each uses its own methodology; some consistent trends emerge but there are also important deviations in findings (Table 3.2). Whilst the Economist data set has not yet been peer reviewed, it has been tested against the IHME and WHO data sets and been found to be sufficiently robust and consonant. We use this data set here as it enables calculation of excess deaths by the territorial blocs we have placed under investigation. According to the Economist, whilst confirmed COVID-19 deaths amounted to 6.4 million in the period January 2020 to June 2022, global excess deaths over the same period amounted to 21.5 million with a 95% confidence interval (CI) setting a range between 14.8 million and 26.2 million (Table 3.2). It is clear that the impact of the pandemic on global health extends much further than confirmed COVID-19 deaths and to confine analysis only to the latter would be to fail to grasp the full extent of the public health crisis.

We now compare excess death rates by country/bloc with the death rates which might be expected in each country/bloc had the global excess deaths total been spread evenly over space, varying only in proportion to population size. Again, we assume countries/blocs reporting excess death rates that (far) exceed expected death rates to be in some way disproportionately burdened by the pandemic and countries/blocs reporting death rates that fall (well) below that which they might expect given their population size to be in some way beneficiaries of the pandemic. On this basis and to the extent that the Economist reports excess data rates which are reliable enough to be instructive, we might conclude that high-income economies now perform better, whilst upper and lower middle-income countries less well. Interestingly, low-income countries continue to escape the worst (Figs. 3.5, 3.6, 3.7, 3.8, and Map 3.4—see also Appendix).

Table 3.2 Estimates of excess deaths, globally and in the UK, various dates, by source

Source of estimate	World			United Kingdom		
	Confirmed COVID-19 deaths	Excess deaths	Ratio of excess deaths to confirmed COVID-19 deaths	Confirmed COVID-19 deaths	Excess deaths	Ratio of excess deaths to confirmed COVID-19 deaths
Economist (January 1, 2020 to December 31, 2021)	5.4 mil	17.8 mil (11.6–21.3 mil)	3.3 (2.1–3.9)	149,007	148,009 (148,009–148,009 mil)	1 (1–1)
Institute for Health Metrics and Evaluation (IHME) (January 1, 2020 to December 31 2021)	5.9 mil	18.2 mil (17.1–19.6 mil)	3.1 (2.9–3.3)	173,000	169,000 (163,000–174,000)	1 (0.9–1.0)
World Health Organisation (WHO) (January 1, 2020 to December 31, 2021)	5.4 mil	14.9 mil (13.3–16.6 mil)	2.8 (2.50–3.00)	158,737	148,897 (133,688–164,445)	0.9 (0.8–1)
Economist (January 1, 2020 to June 30, 2022)	6.4 mil	21.5 mil (14.0–26.2 mil)	3.9 (2.3–4.1)	180,884	154,400 (151.100–161.700)	0.86 (0.84–0.89)

Source Economist coronavirus-excess-deaths-tracker, Institute of Health Metrics and Evaluation, and World Health Organisation

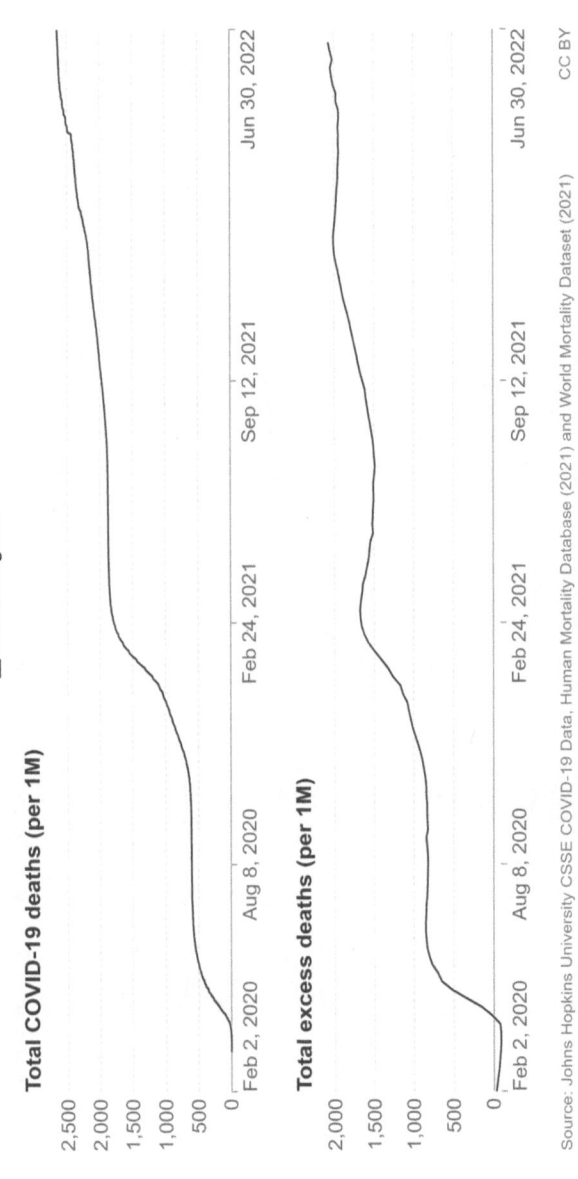

Fig. 3.5 Cumulative confirmed COVID-19 deaths and excess deaths per million, UK January 2020 to June 2022 (*Source* John Hopkins University CSSE COVID-19 Data, Human Mortality Database and World Mortality Database)

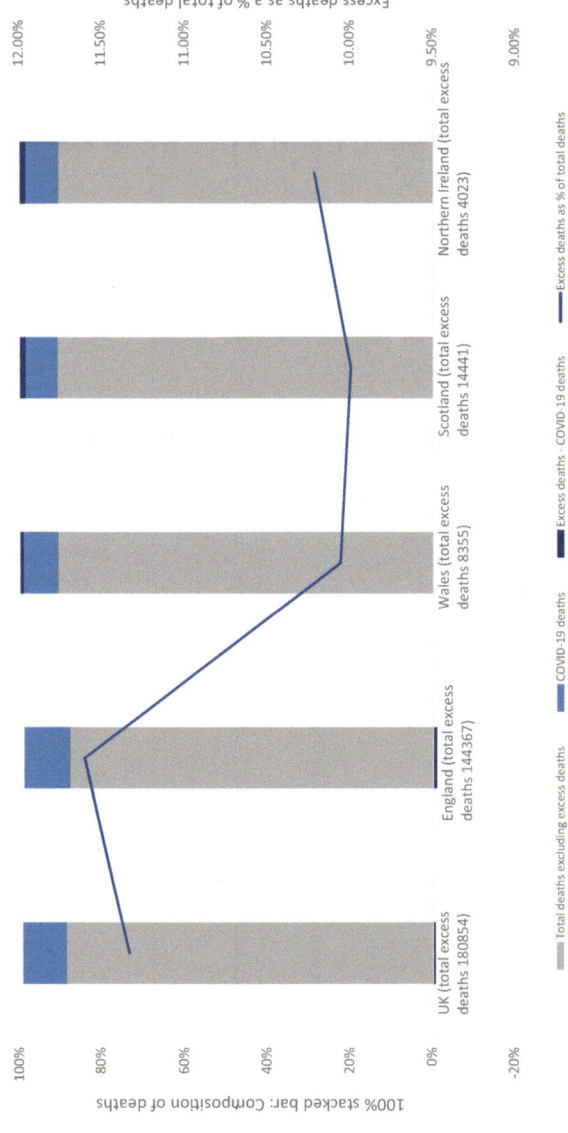

Fig. 3.6 Composition of UK nations' death rates (breakdown in % of total deaths, total deaths excluding COVID-19 deaths, excess deaths and COVID-19 deaths) January 2020 to June 2022 (*Source* ONS [England and Wales], SNR [Scotland] NISRA [N Ireland])

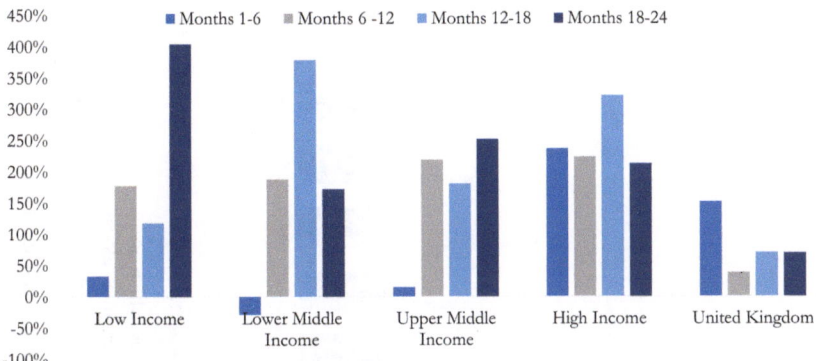

Fig. 3.7 Ratio of actual excess deaths and excess deaths expected had total global excess deaths been distributed according to population size in six month intervals January 2020-December 2021 The United Kingdom in the context of World Bank Income Regions (*Source* World Health Organisation)

Advanced liberal market democracies in global context

- Across the first six months of the pandemic (January to June 2020) most of the Western-leaning territorial blocs we examined endured between 2 and 3 times the excess deaths they might have expected had the disease been evenly distributed according to population size. But thereafter their share of the burden of disease declined and in the first six months of 2022 most emerged with much fewer excess deaths than the global average per capita. The upshot is that across the period January 2020 to June 2022, some advanced liberal market democracies witnessed below average—not above average excess death rates.
- The V-Dem liberal democracies, Economist Democracy Index and CATO/Fraser Human Freedom blocs, and EU27 all secured better than average outcomes. Might this imply that there is no basis upon which to tie liberal freedoms and democracy to poor outcomes? Not especially; the relationship first remains in need of unveiling. The WHO's European Region, high ranking countries in the DHL Global Connectivity Index, the NATO region, the Paris Club bloc,

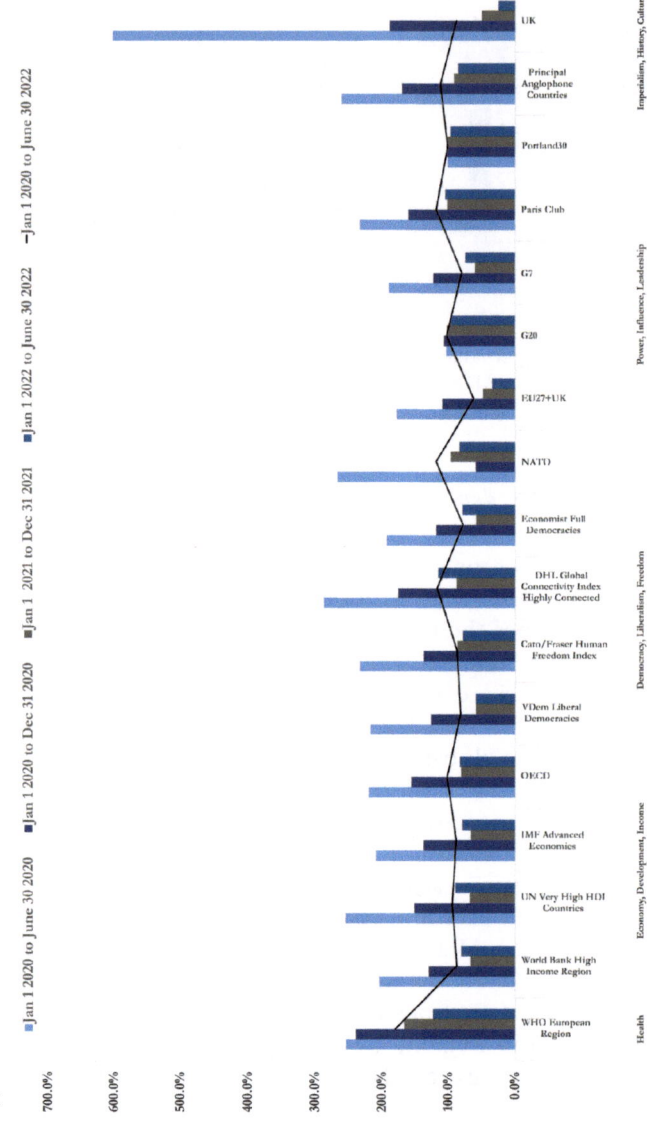

Fig. 3.8 Ratio (in %) of actual % share of excess deaths relative to % share of excess deaths which would have occurred had COVID-19 spread evenly across the earth equally, varying only by population size. **a** Territorial blocs in global context (assumes global excess deaths total is shared across the earth equally, varying only by population size) January 2020–June 2022. **b** UK in the context of various globally significant Western territorial units/blocs (assumes total excess deaths recorded in each bloc are shared across those blocs evenly) January 2020–June 2022 (*Source* John Hopkins CSSE COVID-19 data and Economist coronavirus-excess-deaths-tracker)

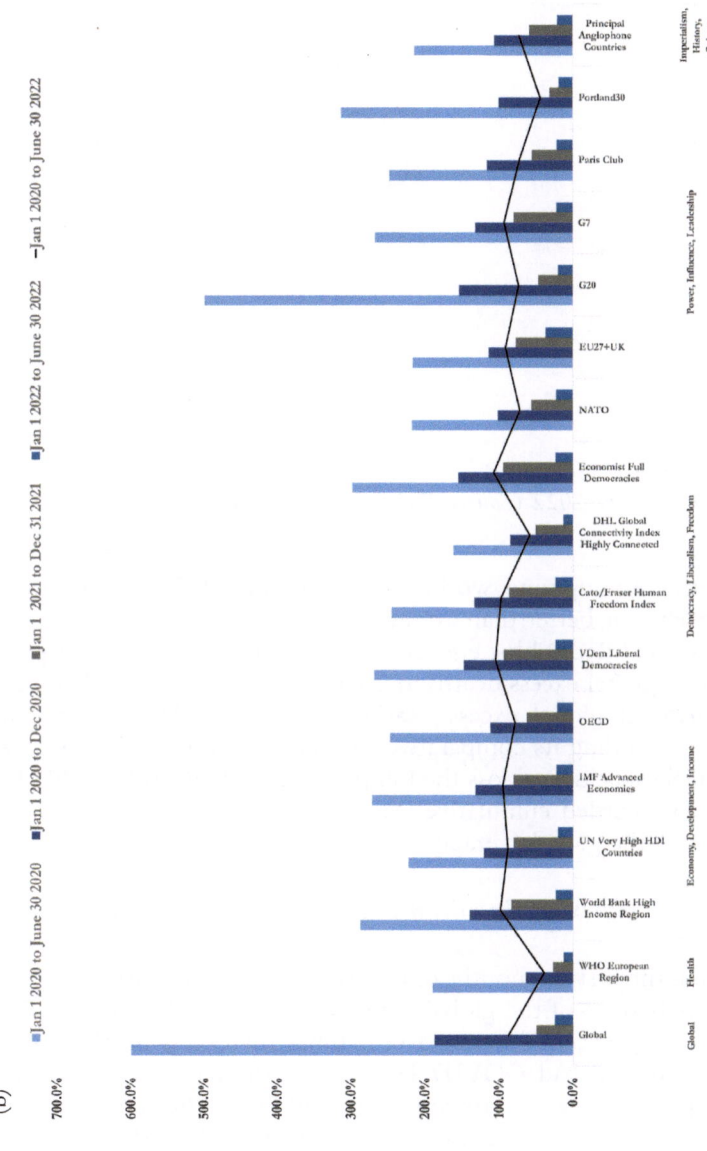

Fig. 3.8 (continued)

Estimated cumulative excess deaths per 100,000 people during COVID-19, Jul 26, 2022

For countries that have not reported all-cause mortality data for a given week, an estimate is shown, with uncertainty interval. If reported data is available, that value only is shown. On the map, only the central estimate is shown.

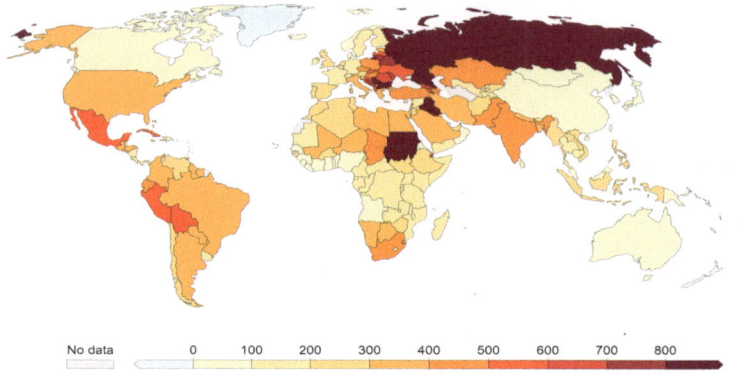

No data   0   100   200   300   400   500   600   700   800

Map 3.4 Estimated cumulative excess deaths per 100,000 people during COVID-19, July 26, 2022 (*Source* The Economist [2022])

and the Anglophone world, all for instance failed to distinguish themselves as better than average.

- Whilst the OECD bloc endured significantly more than its expected share of global excess deaths in 2020, this bloc dramatically reduced its share of global excess deaths from Jan. 2021 onwards. Still, notwithstanding its comparatively superior health, wealth, and institutional capacities, across the full period Jan. 2020 to June 2022 the OECD recorded cumulative excess death rates which were only in line with the global average.

The UK in the context of the advanced liberal market democracies

- During the first six months of the pandemic (January to June 2020), with only 0.8% of the global population, the UK registered 3.5% of the world's excess deaths—over 6 times the excess deaths it might have expected had COVID-19 been distributed evenly over space on a per capita basis. For the entirety of 2020, this figure remained twice the global average rate. Across 2021 it fell further to half the

3 CHASTENED: THE UK'S ENCOUNTER WITH COVID-19 ...   73

global average per capita and in the first six months of 2022 (to June 2022) it bottomed out at only a quarter of the global average rate. The net result is that across the full period of January 2020 to June 2022, the UK registered only 72% of the excess deaths it might have expected.

- When set into the context of the liberal democratic advanced capitalist world, it is evident that the UK has transitioned from being amongst the West's poorest performers in the early months of the pandemic to being one of its best by 2022, comparing especially favourably with the WHO's European Region collective, the OECD and NATO blocs, the high-ranking DHL Global Connectivity Index, and the Anglophone world.

- With respect to the OECD, the UK performed below average across 2020 but has since shown improvement; whilst in the first six months of 2020 the UK recorded 2.7 times the excess deaths per capita recorded across the OECD, in the first six months of 2022 it now shouldered on 0.2 times this bloc's excess deaths rate. Between January 2020 and June 2022, the UK shouldered only 80% of the excess deaths it might have expected if it achieved average OECD outcomes. On June 30, 2020, December 31, 2020, June 30, 2021, December 31, 2021, and June 30, 2022, respectively, amongst OECD member states, the UK was ranked 2/38, 10/38, 14/38, 15/38, 15/38 for excess deaths per capita.

So, what—if anything—might global geographies of excess death rates tell us about the extent of the burden of disease borne by Western liberal market democracies generally and the UK specifically?

Certainly, evolving geographies of excess deaths demand that we temper and qualify conclusions reached on the basis of confirmed cases and deaths. We note that globally, there have been significantly more excess deaths than those confirmed as COVID-19 deaths. Moreover, because the geographical distribution of these excess deaths is significantly different from the geography of confirmed COVID-19 deaths, so too the geography of the public health crisis as a whole needs to be understood as layered and complex. Generally, confirmed COVID-19 deaths account for most excess deaths in the more developed Global North, whilst in the less developed Global South excess deaths extend considerably beyond confirmed COVID-19 deaths. The lower-than-average confirmed

COVID-19 death rates in Africa and Central and Southeast Asia in particular come to be offset and even eclipsed by higher-than-average excess
death rates. In the case of the UK, confirmed COVID-19 deaths account
almost fully for excess deaths (Fig. 3.7). Because the UK had very high
confirmed COVID-19 deaths in the first year of the pandemic, so too
it had a greater-than-average excess deaths. As confirmed COVID-19
deaths fell, so too did the UK's share of excess deaths. Whilst some upper
and lower middle-income countries in Africa and Central and Southeast
Asia have endured growing confirmed COVID-19 deaths, their increased
share of the global burden of disease over time has stemmed from their
greater level of excess deaths (Map 3.5, Fig. 3.9, and Appendix).

A simplistic deduction would be that conclusions predicated upon
confirmed COVID-19 death rates are essentially misleading; they reflect
little more than variegated under-diagnosis arising from spatial variations
in the efficacy of testing, certification, and reporting procedures. Global
North countries and Western leaning global groupings and blocs only
appear to have borne a disproportionate burden of disease because their
data infrastructures are superior. That the gap between estimated excess
deaths and reported COVID-19 deaths is much larger in lower and upper
middle-income countries suggests that the real geography of COVID-19
is skewed much more towards the Global South than has been understood
to date.

In our view, it would be a stretch for the UK to draw much comfort
from this logic.

- It is not yet clear why the gap between confirmed COVID-19 deaths
  and excess deaths is greater in the Global South. Inadequate data
  infrastructure is only one possible explanation. It might well be that
  the geography of officially confirmed COVID-19 deaths is indeed
  an accurate depiction of reality. Excess mortality may arise principally as a product of deferred and reduced healthcare and other
  key services or pandemic-related changes in behaviours (fewer traffic
  accidents, less air pollution, and so on). Perhaps Global North countries, and in particular the UK, have failed to contain COVID-19
  itself but, owing to their superior economic, social, and political
  resources, have been able to stop its downstream, derivative, and
  secondary public health consequences. By dint of their weaker institutional capacities less developed Global South countries may have
  found it more difficult to stem spillover effects and break the link

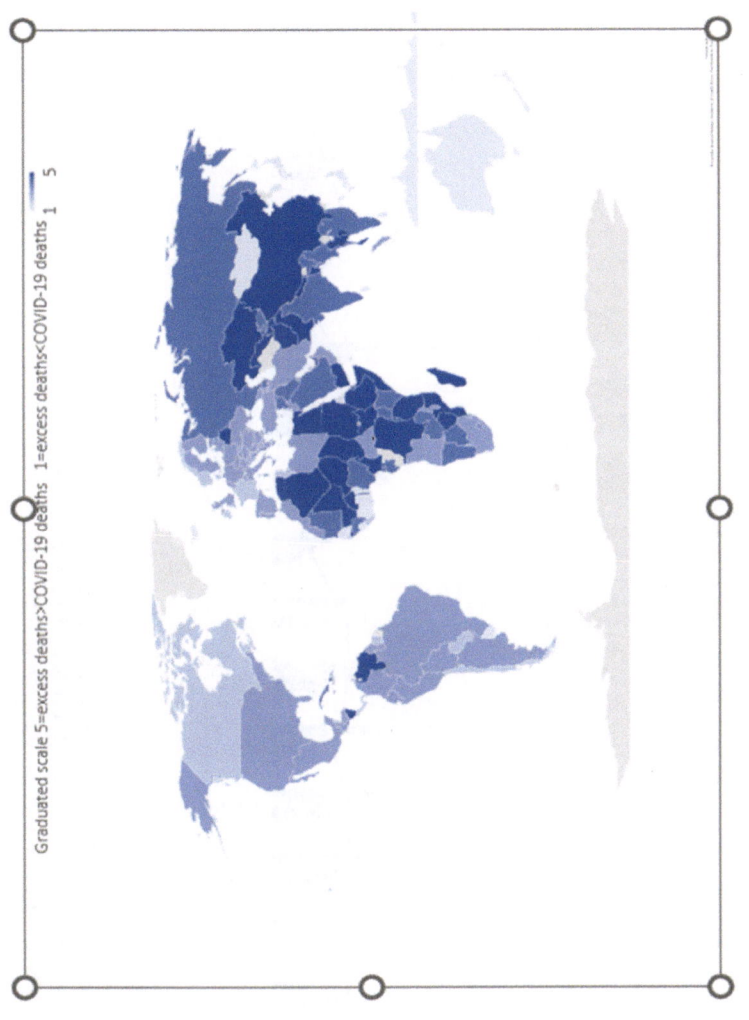

Map 3.5 Ratio of excess deaths to confirmed COVID-19 deaths January 2020 to June 2022 (*Source* John Hopkins CSSE COVID-19 data and Economist coronavirus-excess-deaths-tracker)

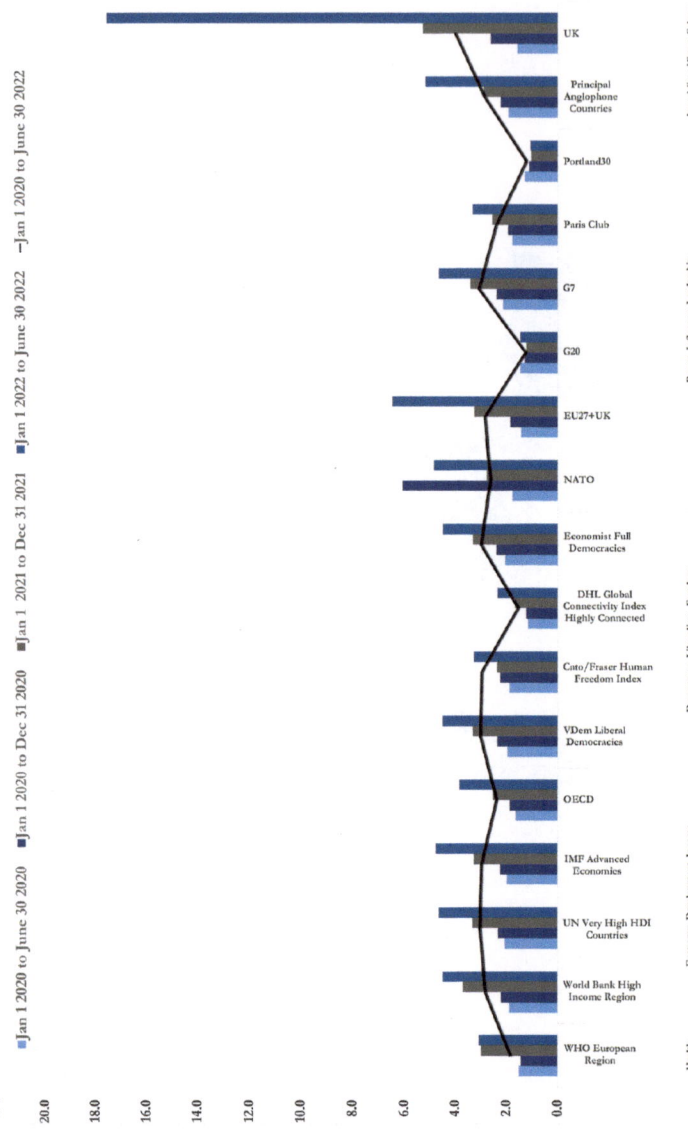

Fig. 3.9 Ratio of % share of COVID-19 deaths and excess deaths—**a** Territorial blocs in global context (share calculated relative to global totals) January 2020–June 2022. **b** UK in the context of various globally significant Western territorial units/blocs (shares calculated by bloc) January 2020–June 2022 (*Source* John Hopkins CSSE COVID-19 data and Economist coronavirus-excess-deaths-tracker)

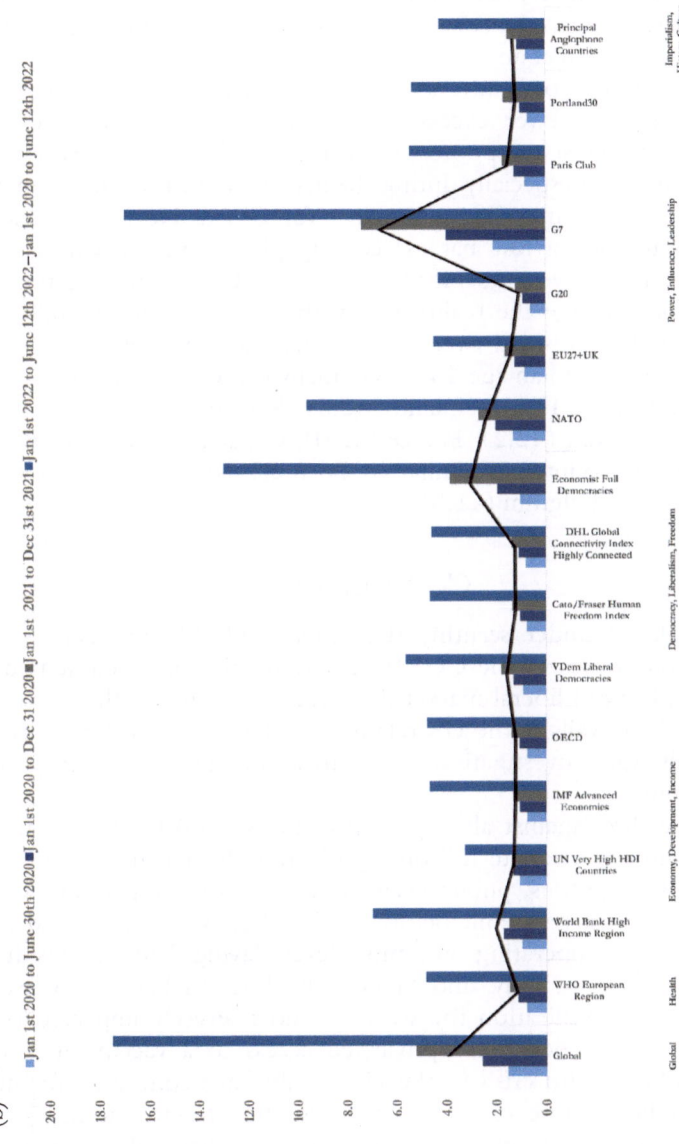

Fig. 3.9 (continued)

between the pandemic and its cascading public health consequences. In these countries, even comparatively modest COVID-19 burdens may have triggered a consequential secondary or downstream public health echo effect and crisis.

- Whilst high-income advanced liberal market democracies may have escaped with fewer excess deaths overall, they nevertheless still ranked amongst the poorest performers during the first year of the pandemic and especially during the first six months of the pandemic. Moreover, we must recognise that for Global North countries to celebrate such a low bar as securing global average excess death rates is itself revealing. Finally, whatever interpretation we prefer, it does not change the reality that with a median age of 40.8 years, the UK has presided over poorer outcomes apropos excess deaths than Japan (median age 48.2), Germany (46.6), Hong Kong (44.8), South Korea (43.6), Finland (42.8), Singapore (42.4), Denmark (42.3), Taiwan (42.2), France (42.0), Canada (41.3), and Norway (39.6) and outcomes similar to Portugal (46.2), the Netherlands (43.2), and Belgium (41.8).

Conclusion

We have placed under scrutiny the global and still emergent spatio-temporal trajectories of the COVID-19 pandemic and documented the travails of advanced liberal market democracies relative to the rest of the world and the travails of the UK relative to other advanced liberal market democracies. Our investigation points to a complex picture that defies cursory summary.

It is true that, against all prior expectations, COVID-19 has indeed exacted a disproportionate toll on high-income liberal market democracies; in these countries, public health outcomes were especially poor in the first year of the pandemic before vaccines became available and when all countries were operating on a more level playing field. Alongside the US, Belgium, Spain, Italy, and France, the UK has been amongst the West's—and by implication the world's—most severely impacted countries. Without the benefit of privileged access to a vaccine it is clear that the public health crisis in the UK would have continued for much longer and been more catastrophic. Only after 12–18 months of the pandemic did the UK meaningfully reduce its share of global deaths and global excess deaths. Moreover, the meaning and implications of the

UK's comparatively lower excess death rate—deaths above and beyond confirmed COVID-19 deaths—are not yet obvious. Whilst now well below average, when viewed across the period January 2020 to June 2022, cumulative excess deaths remain excessively high given the country's economic and institutional strengths. Certainly, across this period cumulative excess deaths per capita continue to be higher in the UK than in the majority of other OECD peers.

Nevertheless, we also underscore the observation that some advanced liberal market democracies and some particularly aggressive neoliberal states clearly performed well throughout the pandemic. Most were able to stop the pandemic from triggering a wider secondary public health crisis and most witnessed much fewer excess deaths. The vast majority secured a lower share of the global burden of COVID-19 deaths and excess deaths over the period January 2020 to June 2022. Poor outcomes were not the sole preserve of the peoples living in high-income 'greying and ageing' Global North; countries predicated upon various political ideologies and bearing a wide range of population pyramids have too been humbled. Over time the hybrid capitalisms of Latin America and the transition states of Eastern Europe have come to rival if not eclipse the high rates of confirmed COVID-19 deaths recorded in OECD member states. And upper and lower middle-income countries in Africa and Asia have yielded to higher rates of confirmed deaths and therefore excess deaths overall. Whilst the global burden of COVID-19 deaths may well have been skewed towards advanced liberal market democracies, the global burden of excess deaths since 2020 have been skewed towards other world regions, rebalancing the overall geography of the public health crisis.

So, what can we conclude? Unless a significant majority of advanced liberal market democracies have simultaneously fallen victim to inept and incompetent leadership, it is clear that COVID-19 appears to be signalling weaknesses and limitations on the West's underlying model of political economy. And these signals would appear to be flashing red in the UK. But acknowledging structural constraints only take us so far. Particular politico-economic-institutional—for us, neoliberal—logics and legacies may have weighed on the capacity of governments to respond to the pandemic, but they have not *determined* the scale, purpose, nor content of such responses. There is no simple line to be drawn between how far a state has embraced neoliberalism, its degree of exposure to COVID-19, the extent of its underlying vulnerability and, the efficaciousness of its response to COVID-19. Although not in conditions of their own choosing, it is actually existing governments that craft public health strategies. Structural conditions create choice architectures, but choices still have to be made.

How the pandemic will end and how many lives it will eventually claim is a question for the future. At the time of writing (July 2022), COVID-19 cases remain very high, and the virus continues to claim a significant number of lives, but deaths (and excess deaths) are showing signs of sustained decline in many places. However, at his weekly press conference on July 12, 2022, WHO Director-General Tedros Adhanom Ghebreyesus sought to warn a complacent world that the COVID-19 pandemic 'is nowhere near over'. In China and New Zealand, a growing chorus of voices is now questioning the long-term efficacy of zero-COVID strategies. Moreover, it now seems (by dint of the rise of new variants) that 'herd immunity' will be an unlikely endpoint. Flare ups, new surges, and perhaps even new waves, are to be expected. Looking to the future, perhaps our most realistic aspiration will be simply the 'downgrading' of the pandemic to a series of periodic and localised endemic outbreaks.

CHAPTER 4

Neoliberalism, Freedom, and the UK's Response to COVID-19

Abstract In this chapter, we go straight to the heart of the matter and consider the implication of ingrained neoliberal norms and logics in the UK government's (comparatively) hesitant and inadequate response to the pandemic. We argue that British neoliberalism's central article of faith—the primacy of freedom as non-interference—has created a hostile environment to effective public health intervention and in consequence a flat-footed and reticent state response to the crisis. By defining freedom strictly in terms of non-interference, and by failing to distinguish between arbitrary and non-arbitrary (and, indeed, freedom promoting) forms of state interference, UK neoliberal policymakers have felt it only natural to postpone and weaken the public health response to COVID-19; resisting necessary interventions until it was too late and lifting necessary interventions at the earliest opportunity.

Keywords UK pandemic response · Freedom as non-interference · Lockdown · Vulnerability · Neo-republicanism · Freedom as non-domination · SAGE

Introduction

In this chapter, we go straight to the heart of the matter and consider the implication of ingrained neoliberal norms and logics in the UK government's (comparatively) hesitant and ineffective response to the pandemic. We argue that whilst undoubtedly aggravated by fallible politicians caught up in overwhelming real-time events and poor decision-making, the UK government's flawed and inchoate response to COVID-19 has deeper roots in the applied political theory that has undergirded the state and its practices for the past forty years. The UK government's deep-rooted and instinctual prejudice against state activism in social and economic life has created a hostile environment to effective public health intervention and in consequence a flat-footed and reticent state response to the crisis. By defining freedom strictly in terms of non-interference, and by failing to distinguish between arbitrary and non-arbitrary (and, indeed, freedom promoting) forms of state interference, neoliberal policymakers have felt it only natural to postpone and weaken the public health response to COVID-19 in the UK; resisting necessary interventions until it was too late and lifting necessary interventions at the earliest opportunity.

Freedom and the UK's COVID-19 Response

Our central provocation is that as a neoliberal idea of freedom as non-interference has become totemic within the British polity, and a foundational assumption for policymaking, it has become ever more difficult to propose and implement activist state policies to improve public health (Entwistle et al., 2016; Salerno et al., 2020). This is the context within which the UK government has fashioned its pandemic response. When defending a particular idea of human freedom comes to trump protecting collective security and public health, the risk is that governments become implicitly comfortable with leaving citizens exposed to vulnerability and precarity. An anxiety that this risk has been badly managed throughout the pandemic haunts the British state.

The British Prime Minister Boris Johnson and the Cabinet of the UK—including but not limited to Chancellor of the Duchy of Lancaster Michael Gove, Home Secretary Priti Patel, Chancellor of the Exchequer Rishi Sunak, Foreign Secretary (and later Deputy Prime Minister) Dominic Raab, and the Secretary of State for Health and Social Care Matt Hancock (and later Sajid Javid, and Steven Barclay) carried final responsibility for fashioning the UK's pandemic response. The Prime Minister deployed the machinery of COBR (Civil Contingencies Committee) to guide the Cabinet's response. In turn, COBR mobilised a sub-committee—SAGE (the scientific advisory group on emergencies), chaired by the Government Chief Scientific Adviser, Sir Patrick Vallance and Chief Medical Officer, Professor Chris Whitty, to solicit independent scientific and technical advice. SAGE itself convened a number of sub groups; arguably the Scientific Pandemic Influenza Group on Modelling (SPI-M) and Scientific Pandemic Influenza Group on Behavioural Science (SPI-B) were the most influential.

Of course, the fragmented architecture of the British state makes matters more complex again. Following the passing of the Coronavirus Act 2020, emergency powers were transferred to devolved governments; in turn, a series of Health Protection (Coronavirus, Restrictions) (England) Regulations were passed in England, Scotland, Wales, and Northern Ireland. Accordingly, whilst aligned and produced in concert, the UK Government (legislating, primarily, for England only), the Scottish Government, the Welsh Government, and the Northern Ireland Executive all fashioned pandemic responses that to varying degrees and at various times deviated. Overall, all four nations increased and decreased the stringency of their closure and containment policies contemporaneously and worked within similar stringency parameters. But at a more granular level, their autonomy and devolved legislative powers periodically manifest some variations in the timing, duration, and stringency of their responses.

To be clear, we do not mean to suggest that the UK Government wilfully abrogated its responsibility to protect lives and livelihoods during the pandemic. Afterall, a series of unprecedented national measures have been introduced at various times throughout the pandemic, including prolonged national lockdowns and mandatory public health edicts, emergency funds for the NHS, higher taxes, and historically unparalleled economic and welfare supports (Bell et al., 2021).

Our argument is that even amidst talk of a Keynesian spasm, we can identify how the neoliberal logic of freedom, defined strictly as non-interference and informing a philosophical presumption against state intervention, remains ingrained in the reflexive instincts of UK policymakers. For the ruling Conservative Party, the pandemic response does not signal a jolt towards a new social democratic dispensation but is instead an aberration, a grudging reaction to an exigency, something to be avoided, limited, and ended at the first opportunity. Accordingly, intervention has often been too little, too late, and too short in duration: a loath concession to the spiralling crisis, rather than a positive, proactive, and pre-emptive intervention (Table 4.1).

Certainly, the language of freedom has been deployed by the government itself routinely throughout the pandemic, casting public health restrictions as a threat to individual liberty.

On February 3, 2020, Boris Johnson dismissed as "bizarre autarkic rhetoric" calls for exceptional public health measures and positioned the UK as "the supercharged champion of the right of the populations of the earth to buy and sell freely among each other". Johnson reasoned; "there is a risk that new diseases such as coronavirus will trigger a panic and a desire for market segregation that go beyond what is medically rational to the point of doing real and unnecessary economic damage....Then, at that moment, humanity will need some government somewhere that is willing at least to make the case powerfully for freedom of exchange". Speaking on the eve of the first lockdown in March 2020, as citizens were advised to stay at home and cafes, pubs, and restaurants were ordered to

Table 4.1 Key dates in UKs programme of national and regional lockdowns

Date	Phase in the lockdown cycle
March-20	First national lockdown announced
May–July 2020	Roadmap out of lockdown, lifting of many, but not all, restrictions
September–October 2020	Restrictions including the 'rule of six' and regional tier lockdown system introduced
November-2020	Second national lockdown announced, presented as a 'firebreak' to stem hospital admissions and ease pressures on the NHS
December-2020	Regional tier lockdown system returns and specific guidelines issued to accommodate the Christmas period
January–March 2021	Third national lockdown announced
March–July 2021	Roadmap out of lockdown, but by now almost all measures removed
December 2021 to February 2022	'Plan B' measures put in place in response to the Omicron variant
February 2022–	Normalisation and transition to 'Living with COVID-19'

Source By the authors

close, the Prime Minister, described the restrictions as going "against the freedom-loving instincts of the British people" (Johnson, 2020a). Again, in September 2020, he lamented that "no British Government would wish to stifle our freedoms in the ways that we have found necessary this year" (Johnson, 2020b). Having reluctantly accepted advice from SAGE to enact a second four week lockdown in November 2020, Johnson was alleged to have retorted that there would be no third lockdown even if bodies might 'pile high'; although the veracity of this allegation remains a matter of controversy and has yet to be clarified. Most vividly of all, the government's plan for ending the third national lockdown was portrayed as a "a one way road to freedom" (Johnson, 2021a), with the Prime Minister urging the public to "take back their freedoms as they can" (Johnson, 2021b) on July 19, 2021 as all restrictions in England were lifted. Indeed, 19th July was widely referred to as "freedom day" in the press and in Parliament, including by the Prime Minister himself (e.g. Hansard, June 30, 2021, col 256).

Lest there be any risk that freedom be (wittingly and/or non-wittingly) sacrificed on the altar of public health, the Conservative establishment acted to ensure that the government would not overstep. Ministers were repeatedly challenged by the lockdown-sceptic Covid Recovery Group (CRG) led by Conservative MPs Mark Harper and Steve Baker, who demanded a 'cost–benefit analysis' to justify the 'necessity and proportionality of each and every restriction'. Sir Graham Brady, chair of the Party's influential 1922 committee and member of the CRG frequently chastised the Prime Minister for affording SAGE a monopoly on advice. Much as the euro-sceptic European Research Group, the CRG garnered enough party support to exert leverage. Editor of the Lancet Richard Horton concludes: "I think that the Prime Minister [Boris Johnson] has been appeasing a small group of MPs, who are vehemently libertarian and anti-lockdown—a group of MPs who simply do not understand the impact of this pandemic on people's lives. And it is the same strategy of appeasement that is used in dealing with Brexit that he's now using to deal with this pandemic. It's entirely political".

History will surely judge the UK government's handling of the pandemic to be painful and woefully inadequate. A 2021 parliamentary report, Coronavirus: Lessons learned to date, refers to government's handling of the early months of the pandemic as constituting "one of the most important public health failures the UK has ever experienced".

In response to concerns over the transparency of SAGE and the independence of the scientific advice it was providing, former Chief Medical Officer Sir David King established a rival group—'Independent SAGE'. This group repeatedly insisted that science supported, if not demanded, that stronger public health measures be taken. For example, in July 2021, the UK looked into a third wave but persisted with 'Freedom Day' and relaxed most restrictions, arguing that vaccines had broken the link between infection and mortality. In an open Letter to the Lancet (Gurdasani et al., 2021), Members of Independent SAGE called this development a 'dangerous and unethical experiment', and called on the government to pause plans to abandon mitigations. Pursuing herd immunity they argued would disproportionately impact unvaccinated children, disrupt education, create a petri-dish for virus mutation, sustain pressure on an already burnt out NHS, and increase the vulnerability of at-risk groups. They concluded: "The Prime Minister's statement today leaves little doubt that the government's latest pandemic plan involves recklessly exposing millions to the acute and long-term impacts of mass infection. We believe this is a terrible mistake".

In his book, *The COVID-19 Catastrophe: What's Gone Wrong and How to Stop It Happening Again,* editor-in-chief of The Lancet, Richard Horton (2020) argues that the UK's 'disastrous encounter with COVID-19' stands as one of the greatest science policy failures in a generation. In their book, *Failures of State: The Inside Story of Britain's Battle with Coronavirus,* award winning investigative journalists for the Sunday Times Jonathan Calvert and George Arbuthnott present a scathing account of the British response, painting a picture of a distracted and out of touch government, holidaying, sleepwalking, and recklessly dithering their way through the pandemic. And even Boris Johnson's own most senior adviser at the height of the coronavirus pandemic, Dominic Cummings, acknowledged in testimony to the House of Commons Health and Social Care Committee and Science and Technology Committee (May 26, 2021) that he and others had fallen 'disastrously short' of what the public should expect and that "when the public needed us most the government failed". Not surprisingly, COVID-19 Bereaved Families for Justice have pushed for a full statutory public inquiry into why the UK government 'serially failed to take reasonable steps to minimise the effects of the pandemic, leading to massive, unnecessary loss of life'.

Those who argue that the UK's pandemic response was too little too late invariably invoke one or more of the following government failures:

- Failure to act on a prior warning (the 'Cygnus' test in 2016) that UK's preparedness for a major flu outbreak was 'not sufficient'.
- Failure of the Prime Minister to chair the first five meetings of COBR in early 2020.
- Failure to fully declare a serious flirtation with the idea of herd immunity in 2020.
- Failure to impose a lockdown earlier in March 2020 and failure to impose a SAGE recommended interim lockdown in October 2022.
- Failure in January and February 2020 to stockpile sufficient PPE, even for frontline healthcare workers.
- Failure to protect vulnerable people in Long Term Care Homes (LTCH)—especially the elderly—and indeed the negligent seeding of the virus into these facilities in March–May 2020.
- Failure to put in place a test and trace system, abandoning early efforts in March only to reinstate the project in April and thereafter (to this day) failing to create a system that was fit for purpose.
- Failure to mandate and enforce the wearing of face masks until late July 2020.
- Failure to quarantine foreign citizens arriving in the UK until June 2020
- Failure to produce a united front by garnering the support of the devolved governments, city mayors, local authorities, and MPs.
- Failure to procure services from the private sector in a competitive way, practising 'chumocracy', and allocating lucrative contracts to companies that failed to deliver.
- Failure to engage the scientific community effectively and failure to heed scientific advice, pandering therein to the idea that SAGE members were part of a politically-motivated cabal.
- Failure to hold a public inquiry amidst the pandemic and therefore failure to learn lessons in real time.
- Failure to convince the British public that political leaders were themselves adhering to COVID-19 lockdown rules, and erosion of trust.
- Failure to suppress death rates in the period July 2021–July 2022, exiting final lockdown earlier than most.

Our argument is that this list of serial failures only partially reflects failed leadership. Given that the sum clearly is greater than the individual parts, it is also a product of the systemic choice architectures that have disposed the UK government to particular policy choices.

On February 13, 2022, as Boris Johnson decided to lift lockdown restrictions for a final time—and a month ahead of schedule, Observer columnist Will Hutton presciently observed:

> *Living with Covid will be an enforced imposition of a particular conception of liberty by the dominant faction of a discredited party – a fundamental misreading of public opinion and the dynamics of pandemic management. It was our new behaviour, as much as state rules, which drove the better-than-expected outcome. We were, in philosopher Isaiah Berlin's famous formulation, practitioners of positive liberty – taking control of our individual destinies through acting together. By contrast, Tory libertarians are really Big Brother imposers of Berlin's negative liberty, defining liberty not in terms of individuals trying to control their life in concert with others but wholly in terms of removing what they describe as coercive state restrictions and obstacles. Concerns about coercion might make arguable sense in some second-order walks of economic and social life – objecting, say, to councils' over-zealous imposition of swingeing parking fines – but in public health issues negative liberty is bonkers. Big Brother removal of safeguards to my good health in the name of individual liberty so that I am free to be made seriously ill by others is as dangerous as any socialist Big Brother....As I have argued in an earlier column, the good society fuses the claims of the 'we' with the needs of the 'I'. Be sure Living with Covid, informed by the bossy negative libertarians of the Tory Covid Recovery Group, will neglect the 'we' almost entirely.....Libertarianism is the new political virus. Immunisation from its baleful effects cannot come too soon.*

A Narration of the UK's Pandemic Response

What policy levers, public health and otherwise, did the UK government deploy to enact its pandemic response? What evidence is there that the UK's pandemic response, when set into global relief, was enacted later, was leaner and lighter, and was terminated at an early stage?

The Oxford COVID-19 Government Response Tracker (OxCGRT) has developed a useful framework and identified associated indicators and metrics through which it is possible to compare and contrast variations in government's pandemic strategies. A Government Stringency Index combines nine public policy domains: school closures; workplace closures; cancellation of public events; restrictions on public gatherings;

closures of public transport; stay-at-home requirements; public information campaigns; restrictions on internal movements; and international travel controls. A Containment and Health Index builds upon these nine indicators by adding testing policy, the extent of contact tracing, requirements to wear face coverings, and policies around vaccine rollout. Finally, an Economic Support Index measures income support and debt relief. The OxCGRT team caution against casual and mechanistic use of these indices, noting that they simply "record the number and strictness of government policies, and should not be interpreted as 'scoring' the appropriateness or effectiveness of a country's response. A higher position in an index does not necessarily mean that a country's response is 'better' than others lower on the index". The indices measure how many of the relevant indicators a government has acted upon, and to what degree but they cannot say whether a government's policy has been implemented effectively. The OxCGRT indices, then, are helpful only if embedded in a compelling interpretive commentary.

Figures 4.1 and 4.2 profile the UK's stringency score in a global context, across the period February 15, 2020–June 30, 2022, whilst Fig. 4.3a–c chart the number of days countries' stringency score exceeded 50, 70, and 90 days, respectively. In many ways, the UK's scale of intervention looks entirely unremarkable. Certainly, the UK appears to be late—even if only by a few critical weeks—in introducing restrictions at the start of the pandemic. From summer 2021, it has relaxed restrictions earlier and faster than many other countries (note: whilst the period from March 2020 to July 2021 witnessed 128,794 confirmed COVID-19 deaths, a further 58,421 confirmed deaths have occurred since July 2021. And, the UK has rarely introduced severely draconian lockdown measures (it has very few days with a stringency score >90). But otherwise, the UK's stringency score appears average and not out of kilter with the majority of its OECD peers. Across the UK's four nations, whilst economic supports and public health measures have presented as broadly consistent, it is clear that lack of coordination has led to some variations in experience (Fig. 4.4). England has witnessed a lighter lockdown in comparison to Scotland and Northern Ireland but differences are marginal when set into global context. Differences principally arise from policy variations apropos the scheduling of school closures, workplace closures, restricting private gatherings, stay-at-home requirements, restricting internal movement, protection of elderly people, and facial coverings policies.

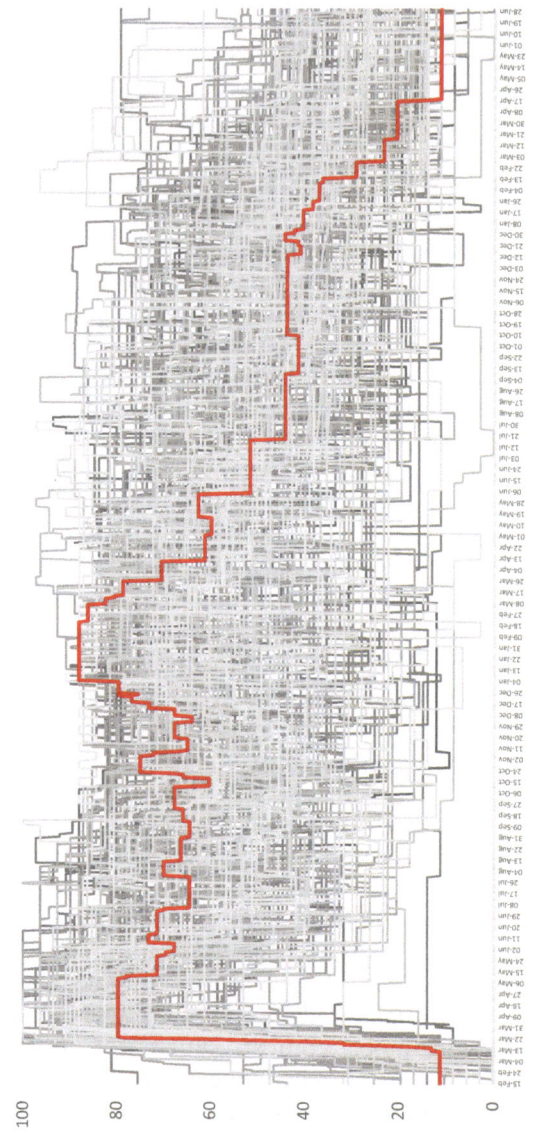

Fig. 4.1 Oxford COVID-19 Government Response Tracker stringency scores by day and for all countries Feb 15 2020 to June 30 2022 (*Source* Hale, Thomas, Sam Webster, Anna Petherick, Toby Phillips, and Beatriz Kira [2020]. Oxford COVID-19 Government Response Tracker, Blavatnik School of Government) (Data use policy: Creative Commons Attribution CC BY standard. NB—UK daily stringency scores by day in RED)

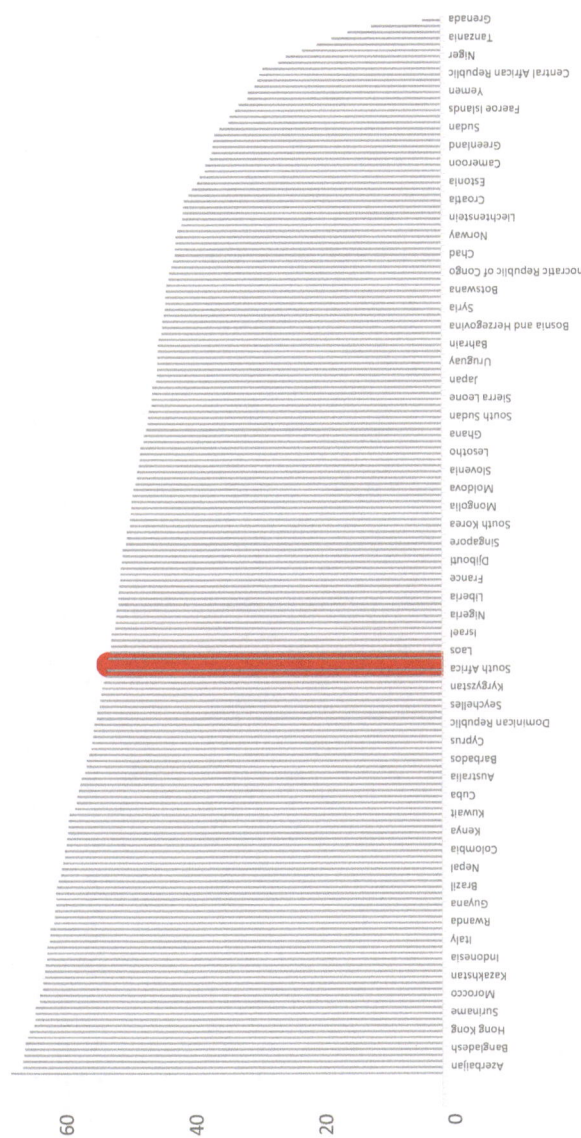

Fig. 4.2 Average stringency scores per day by country Feb 15 2020 to June 30 2022 (*Source* Hale, Thomas, Sam Webster, Anna Petherick, Toby Phillips, and Beatriz Kira [2020]. Oxford COVID-19 Government Response Tracker, Blavatnik School of Government) (Data use policy: Creative Commons Attribution CC BY standard. NB—UK daily stringency by day in RED)

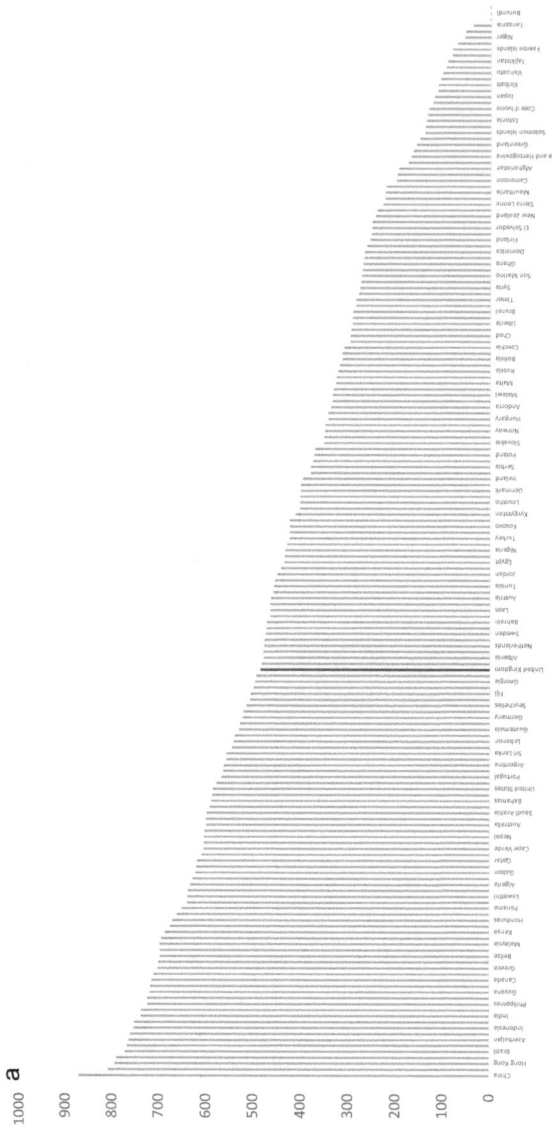

Fig. 4.3 Number of days stringency score >50, 70 and 90 by country February 2020 to June 2022. **a** Number of days with stringency score >50. **b** Number of days with stringency score >70. **c** Number of days with stringency score >90. (*Source* Oxford COVID-19 Government Response Tracker and John Hopkins Coronavirus Resources Centre. NB UK in RED)

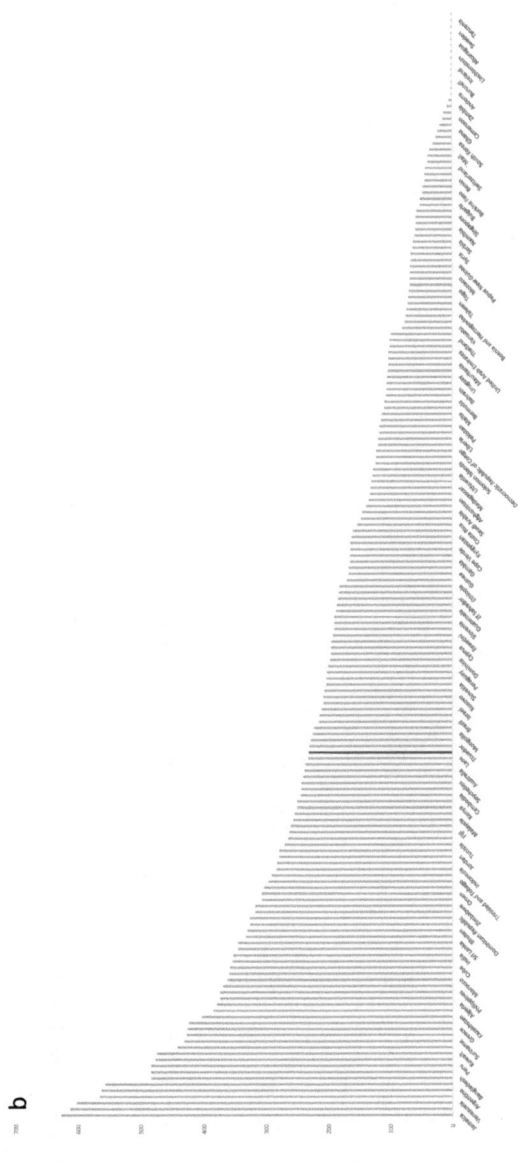

Fig. 4.3 (continued)

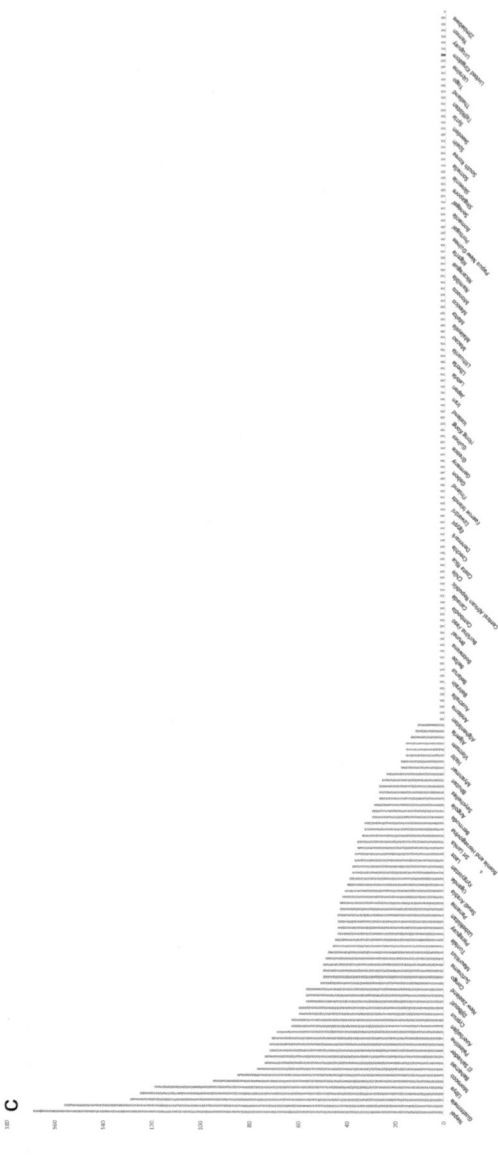

Fig. 4.3 (continued)

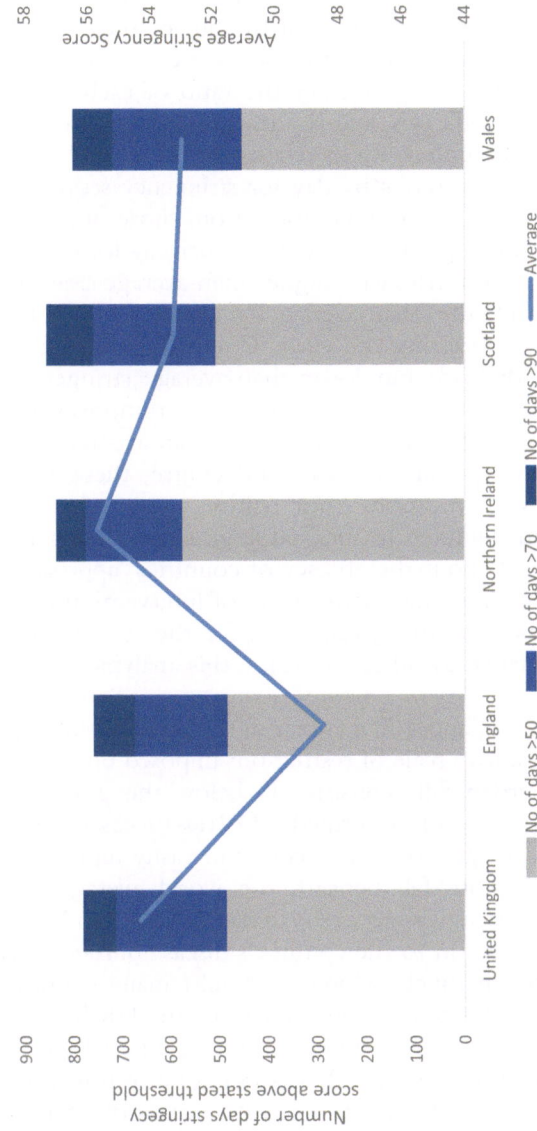

Fig. 4.4 Profile of stringency scores >50, 70 and 90 by UK nation February 2020–June 2022 (*Source* Oxford COVID-19 Government Response Tracker and John Hopkins Coronavirus Resources Centre)

But of course, it is more insightful to examine changes in stringency scores in relation to changes in cases and deaths; countries with low stringency scores may be performing well by dint of their low number of cases and deaths. To calibrate stringency scores relative to disease burdens we calculated for every country the ratio of each of (a) stringency scores, (b) confirmed cases, and (c) deaths per million for each day from March 1, 2020 to June 3, 2022 relative to the global average for that day. We compared the ratios by day for stringency scores for cases (subtracting ratios per country per day for b from those of a) and separately for deaths (subtracting ratios per country per day for c from those of a). We supposed that countries with higher-than-average case and death loads might also have a higher-than-average stringency scores as they seek to regain control by suppressing the virus. Countries with higher-than-average case and death loads but lower-than-average stringency scores may present as less willing to intervene. In contrast countries with lower-than-average case and death loads but higher-than-average stringency scores may present as especially cautious. Of course, these are suppositions—perhaps even provocations—not truths. Comparing ratios can only take us so far and is limited by methodological constraints: certainly, nothing can be inferred about the efficacy of countries' approaches. But if used to gain insights into the relative scale of intervention in the UK in comparison to other countries, calibrated for the severity of disease burdening the UK relative to other countries, this analysis is at the least suggestive.

Figures 4.5a–c, 4.6a–c, and 4.7, summarise the principal findings. Not surprisingly the comparative scale of restrictions imposed on the UK relative to its disease burden falls consistently below the global average. Indeed, relative to its scale of confirmed COVID-19 cases and deaths, the UK has a lower average stringency score and vastly more days when its relative stringency score fell beneath the world average. In other words, whilst the UK's stringency score is in itself average and unremarkable, when viewed in relation to the country's disease burden, it appears proportionately lighter in touch. Moreover, whilst many countries vary greatly in their relative stringency score over time, the UK has witnessed a sustained below average performance, troughing especially in concert with its three principal waves. Whilst deteriorating ratios primarily reflect increases in confirmed COVID-19 and deaths, across the period stringency levels have been lower than they might have been and there has been scope to significantly scale scores.

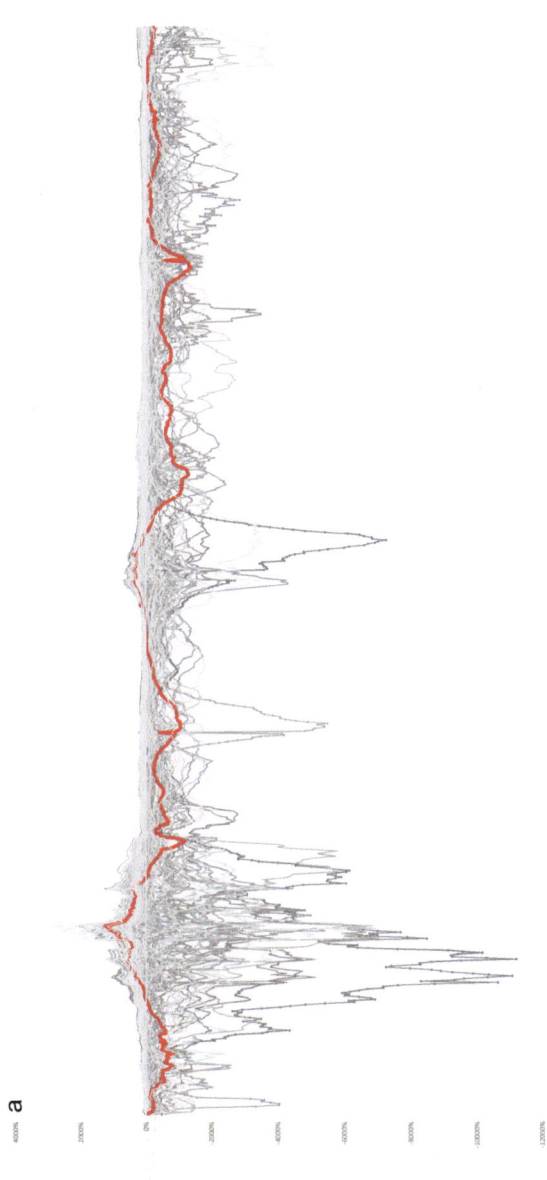

Fig. 4.5 **a** Oxford COVID-19 Government Response Tracker: Relative Stringency Score relative to the number of cases by country by day March 2020–June 2022. **b** Oxford COVID-19 Government Response Tracker: Relative Stringency Score relative to the number of cases by select countries by day March 2020–June 2022. **c** Oxford COVID-19 Government Response Tracker: Number of days stringency score < 0 by country March 2020–June 2022 (*Source* Oxford COVID-19 Government Response Tracker and John Hopkins Coronovirus Resources Centre. NB—UK = RED line)

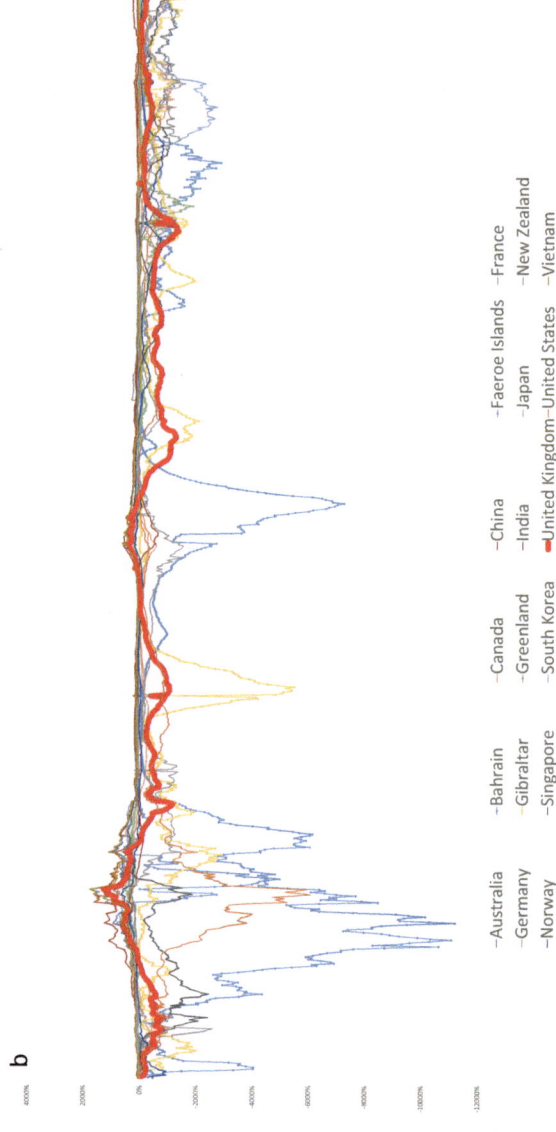

Fig. 4.5 (continued)

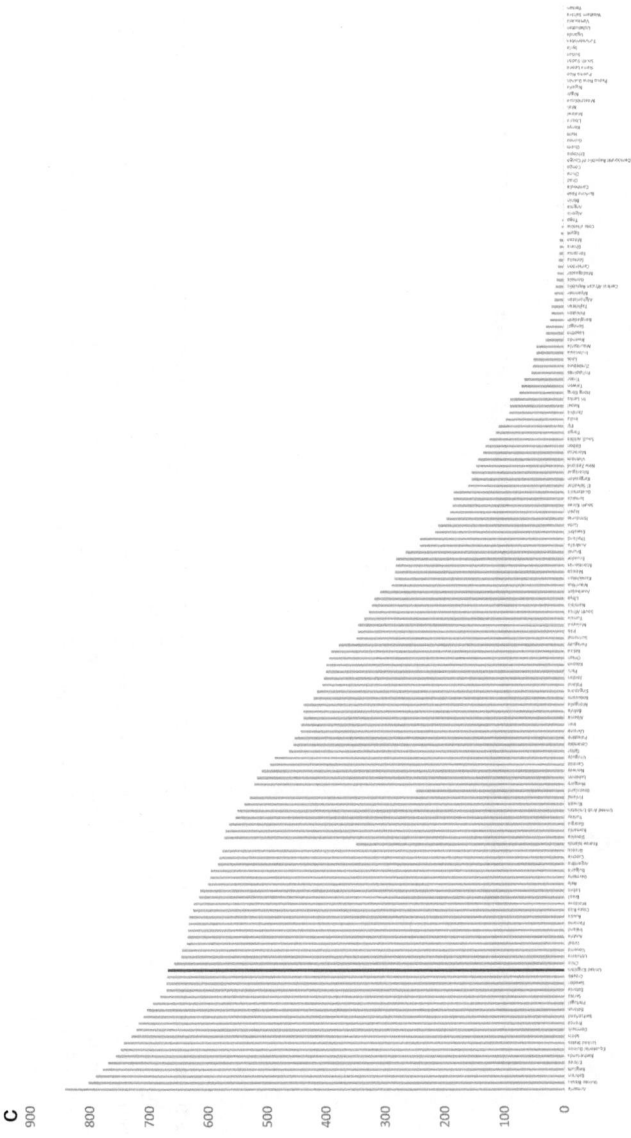

Fig. 4.5 (continued)

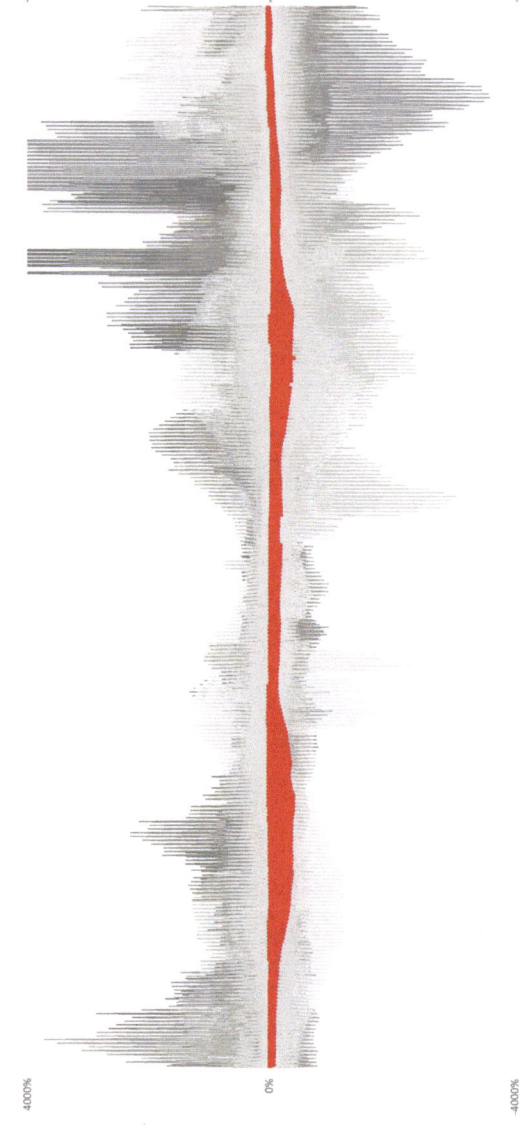

Fig. 4.6 **a** Oxford COVID-19 Government Response Tracker: Relative Stringency Score relative to the number of deaths by country by day March 2020–June 2022. **b** Oxford COVID-19 Government Response Tracker: Relative Stringency Score relative to the number of deaths by country by day March 2020–June 2022. **c** Oxford COVID-19 Government Response Tracker: Number of days ratio of stringency score relative to deaths < 0 by country March 2020–June 2022 (*Source* Oxford COVID-19 Government Response Tracker and John Hopkins Coronovirus Resources Centre. NB—UK = RED line)

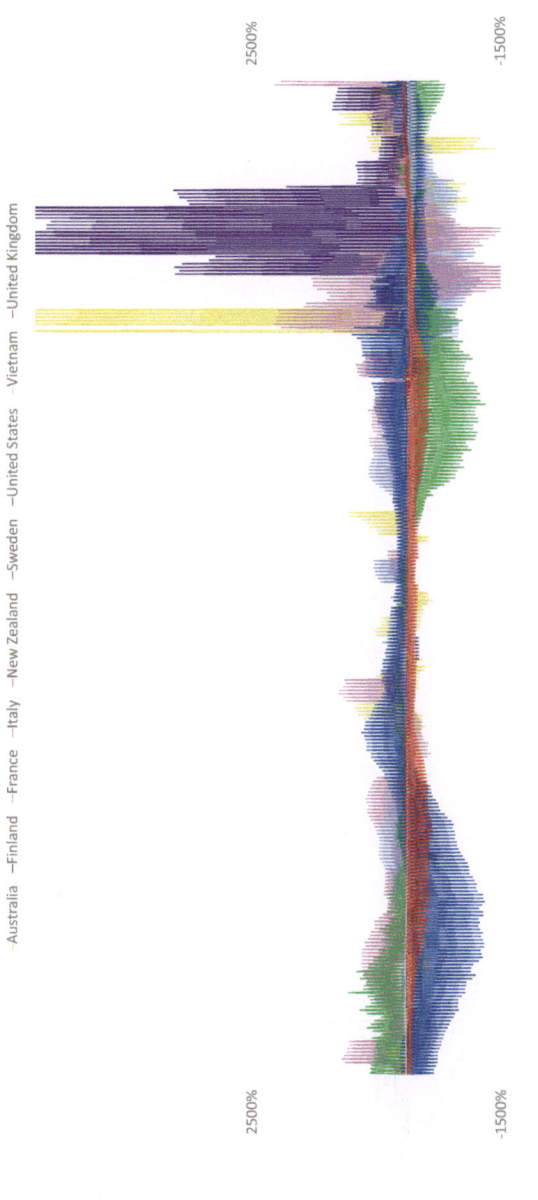

Fig. 4.6 (continued)

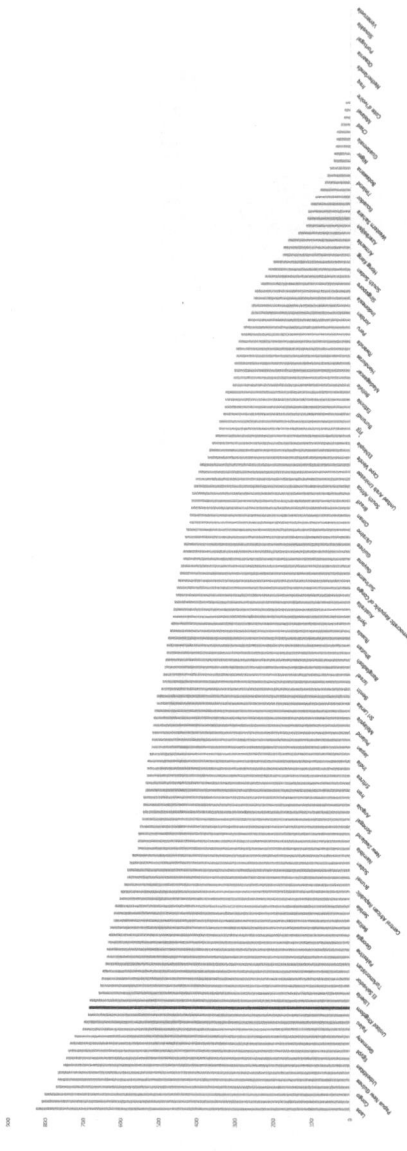

Fig. 4.6 (continued)

Fig. 4.7 The extent to which the UKs relative stringency score fell short of its relative case rate and relative death rate March 2020–June 2022 (*Source* Oxford COVID-19 Government Response Tracker and John Hopkins Coronovirus Resources Centre)

The Oxford COVID-19 Government Response Tracker project has highlighted how the rate at which more measures, such as 'lockdowns', are adopted is critical to addressing the spread of the virus (Hale et al., 2020). New Zealand offers a paradigmatic counter-example to the UK, and reflects international best practice. For example, the New Zealand government began introducing risk-informed border restrictions from February 2, 2020, in advance of World Health Organisation advice and before even the first local case of COVID-19 was confirmed in Auckland on February 28, 2020. Further strategies were subsequently introduced to suppress the virus, with a nationwide lockdown brought into effect on March 25, 2020. This was just twenty-six days after the first case of COVID-19 had been identified and before a single death from the disease had been recorded. Evidence suggests the unprecedented speed and intensity of New Zealand's national response prevented the country facing the scale of epidemic seen in similar high-income countries (Jefferies et al., 2020).

In contrast, the UK's hesitant and reluctant approach towards introducing public health measures appears even more stark. Whilst other governments around the world immediately, or even pre-emptively, introduced increasingly stringent measures to curb the virus as reported cases began to rise, the UK's response can be seen to lag the initial spike in infections (Hale et al., 2020, 11).

After initially introducing an, albeit limited, series of international travel measures from late January 2020 onwards to prevent the spread of COVID-19 cases to the country, the UK withdrew all border measures, including quarantine and self-isolation guidance for new arrivals, between March 13, 2020 and June 8, 2020. Evidence suggests that thousands of new infections may have been brought into the country during this time (Home Affairs Committee, 2020, 3). Meanwhile, the UK's first national 'lockdown'—with people told to stay at home, gatherings banned, and non-essential businesses closed—did not come into full effect until March 26, 2020, almost two months after the first local cases were recorded and when over 1800 people had already died with the virus (Brown & Kirk-Wade, 2021, 6; Gov.uk, n.d.).

By Summer 2020, as the first wave of the pandemic receded in response to the lockdown, social distancing, and self-isolation measures, the UK government began to ease restrictions. Despite no material change to the public health risk posed by COVID-19 (hundreds of cases were still being recorded daily in the UK as restrictions were eased, immunity amongst the population was low, and the rollout of effective vaccines would not begin until December 2020), the government nonetheless encouraged citizens to return to their workplaces, to 'eat out to help out' at local hospitality venues, and relax social distancing practices with friends, family, and colleagues (Institute for Government, 2021). National restrictions were replaced with an often opaque and seemingly arbitrary, 'whack-a-mole' strategy of tiered, local restrictions which subsequently proved inadequate to stem the tide as cases, predictably, began to rise again across the county (Health and Social Care and Science and Technology Committees, 2021, 46–48).

With a second wave of the pandemic beginning to swell, the Government's Scientific Advisory Group for Emergencies (SAGE), advised on September 21, 2020 that a short, sharp 'circuit breaker' lockdown lasting two weeks could help to reduce the spread of the virus. This advice was resisted for more than a month, until 31st October when a second, time-limited national lockdown lasting four weeks was announced by the Prime Minister (Health and Social Care and Science and Technology Committees, 2021, 49–51).

When the second national lockdown came to an end on December 2, 2020, cases still remained high and began to rapidly rise again, driven by the emergence of the significantly more transmissible Alpha variant of the virus. Despite the rapidly worsening situation, the government reverted to reliance on piecemeal local restrictions, including a patchwork of restrictions limiting social gatherings over the Christmas period. A third national lockdown would not be introduced until 6 January 2021, by which point the UK was recording over 50,000 new cases daily (Bell & Brewer, 2021, 8; Brown & Kirk-Wade, 2021, 19; Health and Social Care and Science and Technology Committees, 2021, 51–53). Analysis by the Resolution Foundation think tank suggests that, had the government acted earlier to combat the rising wave of new cases, up to 27,000 deaths could have been prevented in the winter wave of the pandemic (Bell & Brewer, 2021, 8–10). By the time restrictions were fully lifted on July 19, 2021, almost 130,000 deaths linked to COVID-19 had been recorded in the UK during the pandemic (Gov.uk, n.d.).

Nobody is enthusiastic about the prospect of lockdowns or other public health restrictions that significantly impact daily life, and nobody would want to suffer them unless they were necessary. However, in the face of a deadly pandemic, such interventions, at speed and scale *have* proven necessary. Indeed, the UK's chief scientific adviser, Sir Patrick

Vallance has noted that, in terms of measures to combat COVID-19, "you have to go earlier than you think you want to, you have to go harder than you think you want to" (in Sample & Stewart, 2021). But throughout the pandemic, the UK government has followed a course often typified by avoidance and delay (cf. Bell & Brewer, 2021, 7; Health and Social Care and Science and Technology Committees, 2021, 40–50; Scally et al., 2020; Williams et al., 2021, 218–220; etc.); waiting until there was no other option but to impose a stringent lockdown, rather than moving pre-emptively at the earliest opportunity to prevent infections, deaths, and pressure on the National Health Service from spiralling out of control.

This pattern of delay represents more than just ministerial incompetence, negligence, adherence to inadequate scientific advice, or mistaken optimism (though these factors can't be entirely dismissed). It is the predictable consequence of adherence to a particular, neoliberal conception of freedom that resists government intervention in the lives of individuals as a tyrannical and oppressive threat to liberty. If lockdowns, social distancing, and other necessary measures introduced by government to protect public health are assumed to compromise individual freedom as non-interference, we would expect neoliberal policymakers to only ever countenance introducing them, reluctantly, when they feel they have no other option. We would expect neoliberal policymakers to resist authorising such measures until the burden of necessity became unbearable; until they calculate that the trade-off between individual liberty and collective safety is justified by the severity of the circumstances, or the weight of political pressure. Moreover, in order to act, the UK government would have had to overcome significant cognitive dissonance to work against the grain of deeply embedded neoliberal thinking about the roles and responsibilities of the British State, built up over recent decades: that the state ought wherever possible to refrain from intervening in the lives and livelihoods of citizens; indeed, that doing so is vital to protect the freedom of sovereign individuals to choose how best to live their own lives.

This language belies the political philosophical contingency of the UK government's response to the pandemic. Perceiving necessary, albeit extraordinary, and unpleasant, public health measures as in conflict with freedom emphasises the particular philosophical commitment amongst policymakers (both implicitly and explicitly) to a conception of freedom understood as non-interference; and the underlying assumption that government ought to avoid intervening in the lives of individuals.

However, alternative accounts of freedom found within contemporary political theory could allow for a different view, whereby the introduction of emergency public health measures need not be seen as in tension with a commitment to individual liberty.

THE NEOREPUBLICAN THEORY OF FREEDOM AS A PROGENITOR OF COLLECTIVE WELFARE

The idea of freedom as non-interference, that liberty exists in the absence of constraint or coercion by others, is far from objective or universal. Rather, this conception of liberty, promoted vociferously by neoliberals, should be understood as historically and politically contingent. Thomas Hobbes was an early defender of this view in his 1651 book, *Leviathan*, arguing that "Liberty, or FREEDOM, signifieth (properly) the absence of opposition...a FREEMAN, *is he, that in those things, which by his strength and wit he is able to do, is not hindered to do what he has a will to do*" (2008, 139, emphasis in original). For Hobbes, the calculation of freedom is blind to the kind of political system individuals live under: "monarchical, or popular, the freedom is still the same" (ibid., 143). The extent of individual liberty depends only on "the silence of the law" (ibid., 146), or the range within which one can operate without encountering actual external interference by the state. Freedom, on this view, operates on a continuum: "in some places more, in some less; and in some times more, in other times less" (ibid.).

It is this idea of liberty that would later influence early liberals, who sought to make the value of individual freedom compatible with the universalist Enlightenment ideal of equality, the commercial considerations of industrialising market economies, and the context of emerging modern democracies in the eighteenth and nineteenth centuries (MacGilvray, 2011; Pettit, 1997, 45–50; Skinner, 2012, 96). Political questions of freedom became something of a utilitarian calculus, asking what level of state interference, under what conditions, could be justified, with John Stuart Mill, for example describing the topic of his 1859 book, *On Liberty*, to be "the nature and limits of the power which can be legitimately exercised by society over the individual" (2008, 5). As we have seen, within *neoliberal* thinking this calculus would increasingly come to be skewed by a more absolutist approach to freedom as non-interference, where the integrity of one's personal sovereignty ought never to be invaded for the good of others.

However, this liberal approach emerged from, contested with, and later subsumed, an older *republican* tradition of thinking about individual freedom and its political significance (Gourevitch, 2015; MacGilvray, 2011; Pettit, 1997; Skinner, 2012). In discussing the republican tradition, we are not necessarily associating with the particular histories and ideas of certain political parties, or political movements that have adopted the 'republican' mantle around the globe (e.g. the Republican party in the US, Les Républicains in France, the Irish republican movement, or anti-monarchy groups such as Republic in the UK). Instead, we are associating with a longer intellectual tradition within the history of political thought, one which has enjoyed a renaissance in recent decades having been excavated, most notably, by the so-called Cambridge school of intellectual historians, including J.G.A. Pocock (2003) and Quentin Skinner (2012).

As with all traditions of political thought, the republican tradition is far from monolithic and its precise contours and boundaries are often contested and open to interpretation. Indeed, amongst contemporary republican scholarship there are important debates and disagreements about the tradition's lineage to the politics of ancient Athens (e.g. Arendt, 1958, 1963, 1968) or ancient Rome (e.g. Lovett, 2010; Pettit, 1997; Skinner, 2012); about its association with participatory models of democracy or more elite, electoral representation (e.g. McCormick, 2011); about its compatibility with free market economics (e.g. Taylor, 2017) or more radical forms of socialism (e.g. Gourevitch, 2015; Leipold, 2020); and about its capacity to adequately critique social inequalities such as racism and sexism (e.g. Coffee, 2015; Costa, 2013; Laborde, 2008; etc.). In this book, however, we will focus on the most influential and comprehensive articulation of contemporary republican political theory, found in the work of Philip Pettit (especially, 1997, 2012).

Pettit draws particular inspiration from a body of political texts that spans from classical Rome, through the Renaissance, through the English Civil War, and up to the American and French Revolutions. It encapsulates the work of key figures including Cicero, Machiavelli, James Harrington, Algernon Sidney, Montesquieu, Jean-Jacques Rousseau, Joseph Priestley, Thomas Paine, as well as the authors of *Cato's Letters* and the *Federalist Papers* (Pettit, 1997, 19–41). These texts are united by a shared concern with *res publica,* literally "public thing" or "commonwealth" (Lovett & Pettit, 2009, 12), a shared conceptualisation of liberty, and a shared focus on the maintenance of important legal and political institutions (Pettit, 1997, 20).

From this historical literature, Pettit has sought to construct a form of republican political theory, that is relevant, attractive, and practicable in contemporary society. This so-called neorepublicanism:

1. Conceptualises freedom as non-domination, or freedom from subjection to the uncontrolled, arbitrary power of others.
2. Understands this freedom to be legally, politically, and institutionally constituted. Freedom is a civic status: whether you are free or unfree depends upon whether you are a citizen of a suitably republican polity with the necessary architecture in place to promote non-domination. Or, in the words of Quentin Skinner, "it is only possible to be free in a free state" (2012, 60).
3. Recognises the fragility of freedom and its constitutional foundations, and so encourages a vigilant, contestatory form citizenship to protect against the threat of domination (Lovett & Pettit, 2009; Pettit, 1997, 2012).

By appealing to the ideas of Philip Pettit in this book, we do not mean to suggest that neorepublicanism offers the *only* vantage point from which to critique neoliberalism, the UK's handling of COVID-19, or the current trajectories for post-pandemic recovery and renewal. Our position is more modest, suggesting only that neorepublicanism offers one *possible* vantage point from which to highlight the contingency of the neoliberal order, the ideological nature of the UK's pandemic response, and the potential to build a post-neoliberal alternative that remains rooted in a concern for the value of individual liberty. However, it is the pre-eminence of freedom within neorepublican thought that means it is a *particularly good* vantage point from which to challenge neoliberalism on its own terms and reclaim the powerful language of freedom from the association with market fundamentalism it has gained over recent decades. By starting from a conception of freedom as non-domination, rather than non-interference, we will show how the republican tradition opens up possibilities for politics, society, and economics that have been closed during the neoliberal era. We will show how the UK's resilience and responsiveness to the crisis have been unnecessarily corroded through adherence to neoliberal ideology. And we will show how a social democratic alternative to neoliberalism could promote freedom more effectively as we build back better.

So, how exactly is the republican conceptualisation of liberty different to that offered by neoliberals, and what does this mean for our understanding of the way freedom has been deployed throughout the pandemic to inform or explain the UK's response?

FREEDOM AS NON-DOMINATION.

The republican tradition of political thought defines freedom not as non-interference, but as *non-domination*. Philip Pettit argues that domination occurs when an agent—be they an individual or a corporate agent, such as the state—has a capacity to interfere *arbitrarily*, wielding some form of discretionary power over another that can be exercised at will and with impunity (Pettit, 1997, 52–55). Freedom, then, is realised, not in the absence of interference, but in the maintenance of an intersubjective status of non-domination, wherein one is not vulnerable to the arbitrary decisions or actions of some other, more powerful, agent(s). For republicans, this free status must be politically, legally, and institutionally constituted via the maintenance of a suitably republican state, one in which all citizens are reliably insulated against any discretionary power that could be wielded over them by particularly powerful individuals, groups, or, indeed, the state itself. This is why republicans have classically held that "it is only possible to be free in a free state" (Skinner, 2012, 60).

This is distinct from the typical neoliberal account of freedom as non-interference in two important respects. Firstly, it means that one can be made unfree by a relationship of domination even where no *actual* interference ever takes place. It is the *capacity* to interfere arbitrarily, at will and with impunity, that matters for republicans, not whether this capacity is ever utilised detrimentally. This is why, according to the republican view, we are made unfree by the rule of an autocratic dictator even if we, by luck or skill, are able to avoid any actual, direct interference or coercion in our lives. That the dictator has the power, exercised or unexercised, to interfere arbitrarily in our lives, at will and with impunity, means we cannot live a free life of our own. Even in the absence of actual interference, we will be unknowingly invigilated or knowingly intimidated by the dictator's omnipresent power to such an extent that we cannot exercise our own will freely, and will thus live a life on their terms rather than our own (Pettit, 2012, 61).

Secondly, and more importantly for our purposes, the republican view also finds that some interference, providing it is *non-arbitrary*, can be entirely consistent with our enjoyment of individual liberty. According to republican theory, interference is non-arbitrary to the extent that it is forced to track the relevant and avowable interests of those subject to it (Pettit, 1997, 65). In this sense, the interference is not some external constraint on my freedom, but an extension of my own will. The interfering agent is not wielding some discretionary power at will and with impunity, but instead acting with reference to my ideas and interests. This is why, for republicans, the interference associated with the rule of law, coercive taxation, regulatory regimes, and so on are not necessarily abrogative of freedom, so long as this interference is authorised by a democratically legitimate and properly constrained government, for public rather than private ends, and is applied fairly, consistently, and transparently, and in a way that is open to scrutiny and contestation (Pettit, 1997, 65, 174, 183–186).

Such interference may certainly limit the range within which one can exercise their freedom, but it does not compromise freedom in and of itself. As Pettit notes with regard to taxation, this will "restrict the area in which those who are taxed enjoy undominated choice, for it deprives them of certain resources, but that is a much lesser offence than domination itself" (Pettit, 1997, 148–149).

But more than this, we can even say that, to the extent that non-arbitrary forms of state interference—such as the rule of law—help to insulate and empower citizens against domination by powerful social, political, and economic actors, this interference can in fact be *constitutive* of individual liberty. As Pettit explains, "as the antibodies in my blood constitute my immunity to certain diseases, the ordinances of nonarbitrary law under which I live constitute my status as a free, undominated citizen" (Pettit, 2002, 347).

The distinction between arbitrary and non-arbitrary interference is crucial in the context of the COVID-19 pandemic. Specifically, it challenges the assumption that lockdowns and other emergency public health restrictions necessarily pose a threat to individual freedom; that there is some trade-off between individual freedom and collective safety that must be justified above and beyond the immediate epidemiological justifications for intervention. From a republican standpoint, such measures may limit the range in which individuals can enjoy their status as free citizens of a free state—with lockdown measures, in particular, severely constraining the range of actions and decisions available to individuals—but, in so far as these measures represent a form of *non-arbitrary* interference in their lives, the free status of individuals will not have been compromised. Nobody will have been dominated.

Whether or not the public health measures introduced by the UK government during the pandemic have, in fact, represented a form of arbitrary interference is an important question. As we highlighted earlier, the way certain measures, such as the tiered system of local restrictions, have been introduced and implemented by the government have appeared at least somewhat arbitrary, with a perceived lack of transparency and consistency in decision-making. Meanwhile, allegations of flagrant rule-breaking by certain public officials throughout the pandemic further challenge the idea that emergency measures have been applied fairly and consistently at all times. Indeed, we may question the extent to which, constitutionally, the UK represents a suitably republican state, capable of exercising non-arbitrary interference at all.

However, the point we wish to emphasise most strongly here is that, in and of themselves, public health measures are not a threat to individual freedom. Regardless of whether they were in fact introduced arbitrarily or not, these restrictions need not have *necessarily* represented a form of arbitrary interference; of domination. From the republican standpoint, it is not the interference associated with such measures that determines whether or not our freedom is compromised, but the constitutional context in which these measures were authorised, scrutinised, and enforced. Public health measures will only represent a threat to freedom if they are, or could be, introduced and implemented *arbitrarily*, as the product of a dominating relationship between the state and citizens. If we wish to protect the value of individual liberty, our task should not be to resist public measures, and all other forms of state intervention in our lives, *tout court*. It should be to ensure the actions and decisions of government are made non-arbitrary through the introduction and maintenance of suitable constitutional checks and balances that force these actions and decisions to track public and not private interests.

To the extent that lockdowns, social distancing, and other measures are introduced in order to specifically limit the spread of a deadly, infectious virus that threatens the lives and livelihoods of people and communities—the result of a collective interest in promoting the public good and protecting the most vulnerable, rather than some arbitrary whim, personal animus, or casual disregard by public officials—these measures will not necessarily represent a form of domination by the state over individual citizens. Such measures may remain extraordinary and unpleasant to endure, but they will not pose a threat to the free status of citizens if they are introduced fairly, transparently, and in a way that is open to meaningful scrutiny. They will represent the fair rule of law in a free state, not the arbitrary whim of a dominating government.

Moreover, to the extent that public health measures represent the capacity of citizens to mobilise the resources of the state to protect their interests—not least their interest in remaining healthy and alive—the emergency introduction of stringent public health measures to prevent harm during a global pandemic could be considered emblematic, and indeed *constitutive*, of our status as free citizens. In such cases, the government is not acting as a dominating master over citizens but as their servant, working to further the common good and the public interest.

By starting from a republican, rather than neoliberal conception of liberty—where freedom is defined, not as non-interference, but as non-domination—we can see the political contingency of the UK's approach to the COVID-19 pandemic more clearly. Delay, hesitancy, and reluctance to introduce public health measures with sufficient speed and scale to pre-emptively stem the tide of infections and save lives—an approach couched in a concern for the freedom (as non-interference) of citizens—was entirely unnecessary and avoidable. Critically, this flawed approach can plausibly be seen to be as much the product of particular neoliberal norms, assumptions, and philosophical commitments that have been engrained throughout the British state over recent decades, as the incompetence, negligence, or misguided optimism of particular officials within the government. Delay and resistance by the UK government was not an accident, but an entirely predictable continuation of a long-standing and deep-rooted policy agenda concerned with protecting freedom as non-interference and minimising state intervention in the lives of individuals.

Policymakers will always need to weigh up carefully the necessity and justification of introducing stringent public health measures in the emergency context of a global pandemic. However, there is no need to resist such measures, or dismiss them out of hand, in order to preserve individual liberty. Indeed, a concern for freedom could instead lead us to *demand* that public officials take necessary, difficult steps to protect public health in the context of a global pandemic. By adopting a republican account of freedom that does not necessarily baulk at the prospect of (non-arbitrary) interference by the state, no matter how extraordinary, it would have been possible for policymakers in the UK to adopt a more proactive, pre-emptive, and preventative approach to the pandemic, introducing public health measures early and fast in the way that other states, such as New Zealand have shown to be most effective.

CONCLUSION

By defining freedom strictly in terms of non-interference, and by failing to distinguish between arbitrary and non-arbitrary (and, indeed, freedom promoting) forms of interference, neoliberal policymakers have felt obliged to postpone and weaken the public health response to COVID-19 in the UK; resisting necessary interventions until it was too late. This course of action was both politically contingent, and entirely unnecessary, with no inherent need to view public health measures as in critical tension with individual liberty. Only by challenging the neoliberal conceptualisation of freedom, as well as the ways this conceptualisation is normalised in political discourse and actualised in public policy, can we avoid further unnecessary hesitance, reticence, and delay by government in the face of future crises.

REFERENCES

Arendt, H. (1958). *The human condition*. University of Chicago Press.
Arendt, H. (1963). *On revolution*. Viking Press.
Arendt, H. (1968). *Between past and future: Eight exercises in political thought*. Viking Press.
Bell, T., & Brewer, M. (2021). *The 12-month stretch: Where the government has delivered—and where it has failed—during the Covid-19 crisis*. Resolution Foundation.
Bell, T., et al. (2021). *The Boris budget: Resolution Foundation analysis of autumn budget and spending review 2021*. Resolution Foundation.
Brown, J., & Kirk-Wade, E. (2021). *Coronavirus: A history of English lockdown laws* (House of Commons Library Briefing Paper no. 9068). House of Commons Library.
Coffee, A. M. S. J. (2015). Two spheres of domination: Republican theory, social norms and the insufficiency of negative freedom. *Contemporary Political Theory, 14*(1), 45–62.

Costa, M. (2013). Is Neo-republicanism bad for women? *Hypatia, 28*(4), 921–936.

Entwistle, V., Carter, S., & Little, M. (2016). Defending public health against 'nanny state' accusations: We need to talk about freedom. https://chpi.org.uk/blog/defending-public-health-nanny-state-accusations-need-talk-freedom/. Accessed 2 May 2022.

Gourevitch, A. (2015). *From slavery to cooperative commonwealth: Labor and republican liberty in the nineteenth century*. Cambridge University Press.

Gov.uk. (n.d.). Coronavirus (COVID-19) in the UK. https://coronavirus.data.gov.uk/. Accessed 28 Dec 2021.

Gurdasani, D., Drury, J., Greenhalgh, T., et al. (2021). Correspondence mass infection is not an option: We must do more to protect our young. *Lancet, 398*(10297), 297–298. https://doi.org/10.1016/S0140-6736(21)01589-0

Hale, T., et al. (2020). *Variation in government responses to COVID-19* (BSG Working Paper Series, 2020/032), pp. 1–29.

Hansard, H. C. (2021, June 30). Deb (vol. 698, col. 256).

Health and Social Care and Science and Technology Committees. (2021). *Coronavirus: Lessons learned to date* (HC 2021–22, 92). House of Commons.

Hobbes, T. (2008). *Leviathan*. Oxford University Press.

Home Affairs Committee. (2020). *Home office preparedness for COVID-19 (coronavirus): Management of the borders* (HC 2019–21, 563). House of Commons.

Horton, R. (2020). *The COVID-19 catastrophe: What's gone wrong and how to stop it happening again*. Polity Press.

Institute for Government [IfG]. (2021). Timeline of UK coronavirus lockdowns, March 2020 to March 2021. https://www.instituteforgovernment.org.uk/sites/default/files/timeline-lockdown-web.pdf. Accessed 28 Dec 2021.

Jefferies, S., et al. (2020). COVID-19 in New Zealand and the impact of the national response: A descriptive epidemiological study. *Lancet Public Health, 5*, e612–e623.

Johnson, B. (2020a, March 20). Prime Minister's statement on coronavirus (COVID-19). https://www.gov.uk/government/speeches/pm-statement-on-coronavirus-20-march-2020. Accessed 28 Dec 2021.

Johnson, B. (2020b, September 22). PM Commons statement on coronavirus. https://www.gov.uk/government/speeches/pm-commons-statement-on-coronavirus-22-september-2020. Accessed 28 Dec 2021.

Johnson, B. (2021a, February 22). PM statement to the House of Commons on roadmap for easing lockdown restrictions in England. https://www.gov.uk/government/speeches/pm-statement-to-the-house-of-commons-on-roadmap-for-easing-lockdown-restrictions-in-england-22-february-2021. Accessed 28 Dec 2021.

Johnson, B. (2021b, July 19). PM statement at coronavirus press conference. https://www.gov.uk/government/speeches/pm-statement-at-coronavirus-press-conference-19-july-2021. Accessed 28 Dec 2021.

Laborde, C. (2008). *Critical republicanism: The Hijab controversy and political philosophy*. Oxford University Press.

Leipold, B. (2020). Marx's social republic: Radical republicanism and the political institutions of socialism. In B. Leipold, K. Nabulsi & S. White (Eds.), *Radical republicanism: Recovering the tradition's popular heritage* (pp. 172–193). Oxford University Press.

Lovett, F. (2010). *A general theory of domination*. Oxford University Press.

Lovett, F., & Pettit, P. (2009). Neorepublicanism: A normative and institutional research program. *Annual Review of Political Science, 12*(1), 11–29.

MacGilvray, E. (2011). *The invention of market freedom*. Cambridge University Press.

McCormick, J. P. (2011). *Machiavellian democracy*. Cambridge University Press.

Mill, J. S. (2008). *On liberty and other essays*. Oxford University Press.

Pettit, P. (1997). *Republicanism: A theory of freedom and government*. Oxford University Press.

Pettit, P. (2002). Keeping republican freedom simple: On a difference with Quentin Skinner. *Political Theory, 30*(3), 339–356.

Pettit, P. (2012). *On the people's terms: A republican theory and model of democracy*. Cambridge University Press.

Pocock, J. G. A. (2003). *The machiavellian moment*. Princeton University Press.

Salerno, M., Hyseni, L., Bickerstaffe, H., Capwell, S., & Lloyd-Williams, F. (2020). OP61 Media analysis of the term 'Nanny State' in UK print and online newspapers: Implications for public health advocacy. *Journal of Epidemiology & Community Health, 74*(1), A29.

Sample, I., & Stewart, H. (2021). Bring in measures soon or risk 7,000 daily Covid hospitalisations. *Sage warns*. https://www.theguardian.com/world/2021/sep/14/bring-in-measures-soon-or-risk-7000-daily-covid-cases-sage-warns. Accessed 28 Dec 2021.

Scally, G., Jacobsen, B., & Abbasi, K. (2020). The UK's public health response to covid-19. https://www.bmj.com/content/369/bmj.m1932. Accessed 28 Dec 2021.

Skinner, Q. (2012). *Liberty before liberalism*. Cambridge University Press.

Taylor, R. S. (2017). *Exit left: Markets and mobility in republican thought*. Oxford University Press.

Williams, G. A., Rajan, R., & Cylus, J. D. (2021). Covid-19 in the United Kingdom: How austerity and a loss of state capacity undermined the crisis response. In S. L. Greer, E. J. King, E. M. da Fonseca, & A. Peralta-Santos (Eds.), *Coronavirus politics: The comparative politics and policy of COVID-19* (pp. 215–234). University of Michigan Press.

CHAPTER 5

Reticent and Hesitant: The Neoliberal State

Abstract COVID-19 points to the critical role of proactive state intervention in response to crisis: the capacity to utilise the power and potential of state infrastructure to protect the public from unnecessary harm. In the neoliberal era, however, the idea that the state can be a positive and legitimate actor in the lives of citizens has been critically eroded. In this chapter, we will show how this neoliberal approach to thinking about the legitimate power and potential of the state weakened state capacity in the decades before the pandemic, constrained the ambition and dynamism of the state during the pandemic, and subsequently left UK citizens disproportionately vulnerable to COVID-19 and its impacts on lives and livelihoods. Whilst it would be incorrect to argue that the British state has been entirely impotent in response to the pandemic, a neoliberal presumption against state interference helps to explain why the UK response to a fast-evolving health crisis has often been partial and limited, granting extraordinary responsibility to the private sector rather than rebuilding state capacity and extending its latitude for effective, proactive intervention in the public interest.

Keywords UK government · Small state · Local government · Austerity · Social democracy · Welfare · Fiscal conservatism

M. Boyle et al., *COVID-19 and the Case Against Neoliberalism*,
https://doi.org/10.1007/978-3-031-18935-7_5

Introduction

On 5th March 2020, the World Health Organisation Director-General, Tedros Adhanom Ghebreyesus called for member states to launch a whole-government approach to the accelerating COVID-19 crisis:

> *This epidemic can be pushed back, but only with a collective, coordinated and comprehensive approach that engages the entire machinery of government... not just the health ministry – security, diplomacy, finance, commerce, transport, trade, information and more – the whole government should be involved... If countries act aggressively to find, isolate and treat cases, and to trace every contact, they can change the trajectory of this epidemic. If we take the approach that there's nothing we can do, that will quickly become a self-fulfilling prophecy* (WHO, 2020).

This rallying cry emphasises the critical role of proactive state intervention in response to crisis: the capacity to utilise the power and potential of state infrastructure to protect the public from unnecessary harm.

In the neoliberal era, however, the idea that the state can be a positive and legitimate actor in the lives of citizens has been critically eroded. In order to promote freedom as non-interference, it has been argued that only a minimal state can be justified, one that limits its intervention in people's lives as much as possible. In this chapter, we will show how this neoliberal approach to thinking about the legitimate power and potential of the state weakened state capacity in the decades before the pandemic, constrained the ambition and dynamism of the state during the pandemic, and subsequently left UK citizens disproportionately vulnerable to COVID-19 and its impact on lives and livelihoods. Whilst it would be incorrect to argue that the British state has been impotent in response to the pandemic, a neoliberal presumption against state interference helps to explain why the UK response to a fast-evolving health crisis has often been partial and limited, granting extraordinary responsibility to the private sector rather than rebuilding state capacity and extending its latitude for effective, proactive intervention in the public interest.

Neoliberalism: Rolling Back and Rolling Out

As we saw in the previous chapter, the commitment to freedom as non-interference has implications for how neoliberals conceptualise the appropriate relationship between the state and citizens, whereby the state ought to minimise the interference that it inflicts on sovereign individuals. This idea also underpins a broader normative theory of the state, its roles, responsibilities, and, in particular, its relationship with the market.

For neoliberals, markets are essential for freedom, prosperity, and the efficient distribution of resources (e.g. see Harvey, 2005, 64; Mudge, 2008, 706; Munck, 2005, 61; Vallier, 2021; etc.). They are the sphere in which sovereign individuals exercise their untrammelled agency to trade, exchange, and live their lives as they see fit. Intervention by the state, in contrast, is seen to upset this, threatening the rationality, efficiency, and liberty offered by free, open, and widespread markets (Munck, 2005, 61). Just as the state ought not unnecessarily to interfere in the lives of individuals, so must it refrain from interfering unnecessarily in the free, fair, and efficient function of the market, or the outcomes of market exchange. As the sociologist Stephanie Lee Mudge states, "Neo-liberalism is distinctive…in its drive to break the 'market' loose in conceptual terms and elevate it to a level above politics—that is, to free it from political interventions of any kind" (2008, 715). The roles and responsibilities of the state must therefore be kept to a minimum, serving only to uphold and safeguard the institutional frameworks necessary for market practices to function properly, and, when necessary, to open new markets in areas where they did not exist previously (Harvey, 2005, 2).

Again, the normative theory of the state adopted by neoliberals, and the logic that only a minimal state is permissible, echoes libertarian arguments made by Nozick in Anarchy, State, and Utopia. As we have already seen, Nozick argues that our natural right to self-ownership means that the state should refrain from interfering in the lives, choices, and actions of citizens. As such, it would be wrong, Nozick argues, for the state to prevent "capitalist acts between consenting adults" (1974, 163), such as exchanging resources or entering into a voluntary contract. Nor should the state seek to redistribute resources according to some favoured ideal of justice. As Nozick explains, this would require the state to "continually interfere to stop people from transferring resources as they wish to, or…to take from some persons resources that others for some reason chose to transfer to them" (ibid.). Whilst states impose and coerce, markets, on the other hand, are considered the neutral products of individual agency; the just outcomes of just processes of acquisition and transfer, that both respect and exemplify the natural rights and liberties of individuals (ibid., 152, 163–164). For Nozick, freedom from interference in the market will therefore always trump the potential benefits of intervention by the state.

No matter how benign or paternalistic the interference, this will always threaten individual liberty, and the way this is mediated by markets and through free exchange.

For this reason, Nozick argues that only a minimal state—one that is "limited to the narrow functions of protection against force, theft, fraud, enforcement of contracts, and so on" (1974, ix)—can be justified. Any state more extensive than that necessary to manage free and fair market exchange—and, in particular, any state that plays an active role in the economy, its function, and its outcomes—would exercise forms of unjustifiable interference and coercion that violate individuals' natural liberties.

This logic, that only a minimal state is consistent with individual liberty, informs a neoliberal policy programme governing the relationship between the state and the market. Neoliberals reject policies that see the state itself playing an active role in shaping the economy and its outcomes, with a preference instead for policies that abdicate more responsibility to the private sector and the forces of free market competition. In particular, neoliberals support the deregulation of markets, the reduction of public spending, the dismantlement of redistributive welfare states, as well as the privatisation of public assets, services and nationalised industries (Hall, 2011, 10; Harvey, 2005, Mudge, 2008, 704–705; Munck, 2005, 63; Vallier, 2021). To be clear, this is not to suggest that neoliberals promote a completely laissez-faire approach towards the market. Instead, they seek to modify and reconfigure the relationship of the state to the market, emphasising the capacity of the state to support, expand, and create free markets rather than control them (Berry, 2019, 608–609; Munck, 2005, 63).

The legacy of this neoliberal approach to thinking about the state, and its relationship to the market, can be seen clearly in the policy agendas of British governments over recent decades. Particularly stark in the UK is the way that, through privatisation and public spending cuts, the state has minimised both its willingness and capacity to intervene purposefully in the economy, and wider society. Multiple levers for action and influence, along with the institutional memory necessary to utilise them effectively, have been lost as the public realm has been steadily sold off and eroded. Meanwhile, public needs and necessities have come to be increasingly served by the private sector, with the British state displaying an instinctive preference for, and reliance upon, market solutions.

Although the UK government spends around the average OECD government expenditure (both as a % of GDP and per capita) the rate of growth in public expenditure has been well below the OECD average in recent years (Figs. 5.1 and 5.2). Meanwhile, local government has witnessed savage budget declines across the past decade, as successive Conservative governments have enacted a raft of austerity policies in the years since 2010 (Figs. 5.2 and 5.3). The overall size of the public sector workforce shrunk markedly across the decade from 2008 to 2019 (by headcount and FTE). Central government witnessed some growth during this period but again austerity has, since 2010, eviscerated local authorities, greatly reducing the capacity of many councils to provide even the most basic of public services (Figs. 5.4a and 5.4b). The consequence of these cuts has been to further centralise meaningful political and fiscal power at the national level, with the UK remaining one of the most centralised of the OECD states despite recent experiments with regional devolution (Fig. 5.5). Not surprisingly, the upshot has been a decline in public trust in government and denuded confidence in the efficacy of the state to represent their interests (Fig. 5.6).

Breaking with a post-war consensus that saw many of the 'commanding heights' of British industry nationalised, the UK has since enthusiastically embraced privatisation. Since the 1980s, a wide array of publicly owned assets, utilities and companies have been privatised, creating new markets where previously nationalised firms or the broader public sector would have operated more or less as a monopoly. Major utilities such as British Telecom, British Gas, as well as regional electricity and water companies were sold off in the 1980s and 1990s, along with public services such as British Rail, and publicly owned companies such as Jaguar Cars, Rolls Royce, and British Airways. More recently, this process of privatisation has continued with the sale of Royal Mail in 2013. Meanwhile, privatisation of state functions has also been facilitated through the introduction of 'Public Private Partnerships' and other forms of outsourcing, whereby private sector firms are contracted to deliver services on behalf of the state. Such partnerships can often enable the private ownership of capital assets, such as schools and hospitals, which would previously have been owned and operated directly by the state (Arestis & Sawyer, 2005, 199–201; Rhodes et al., 2014). The National Audit Office estimated in 2013 that around half of all UK government expenditure on goods and services was now through outsourcing to the private sector (NAO, 2013, 10). Such forms of privatisation exemplify the steady shift away from direct

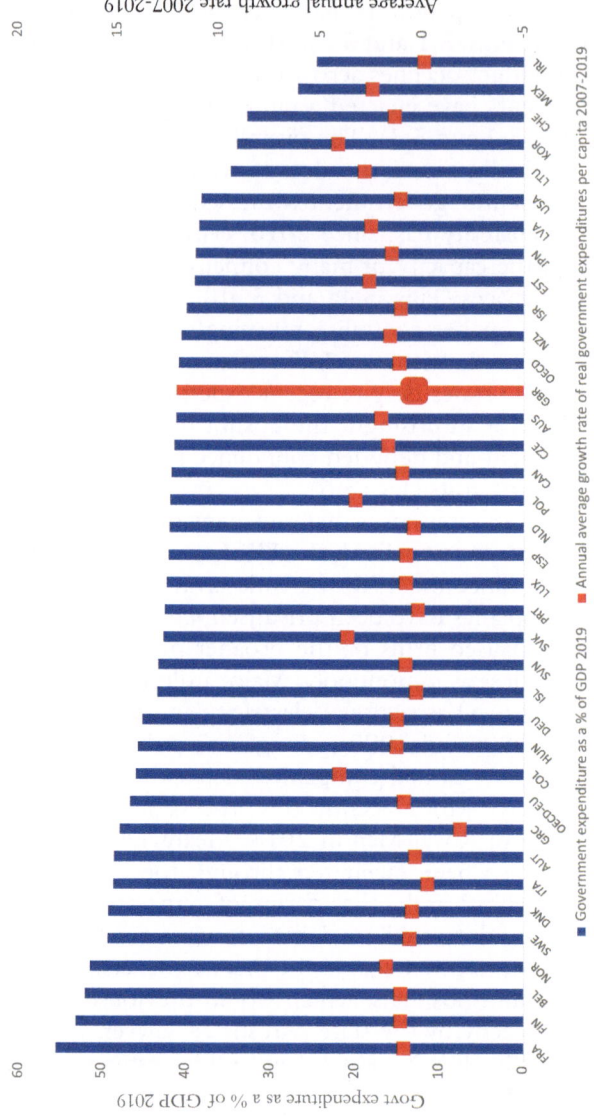

Fig. 5.1 Government expenditure as a % of GDP 2019 and annual average growth rate of real government expenditures per capita, 2007–2019 (*Source* OECD Government at a glance, 2021)

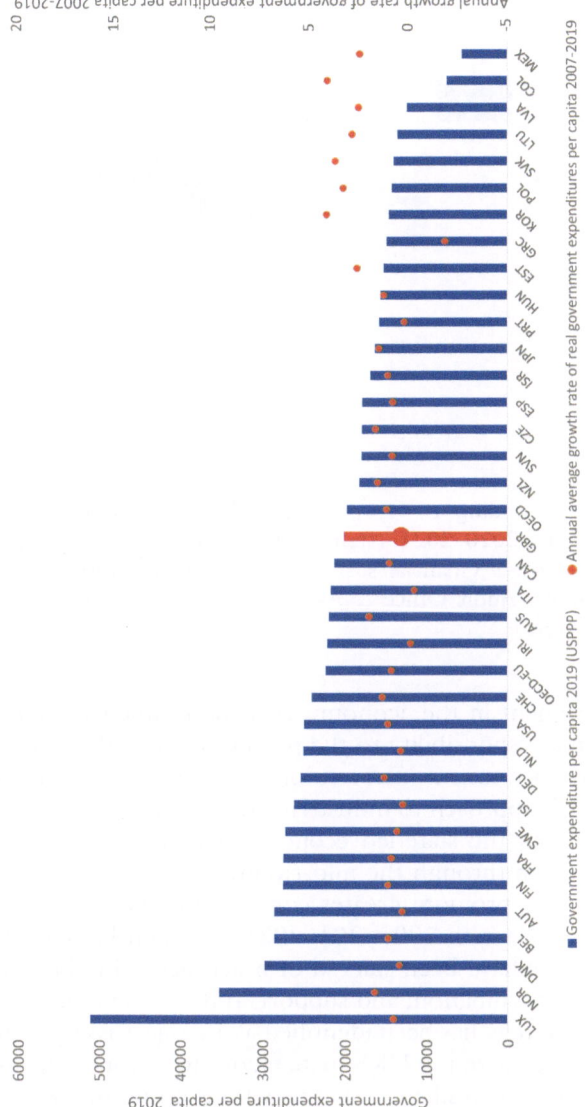

Fig. 5.2 Government expenditure per capita 2019 (USPPP) and annual average growth rate of real government expenditures per capita, 2007–2019 (*Source* OECD Government at a glance, 2021)

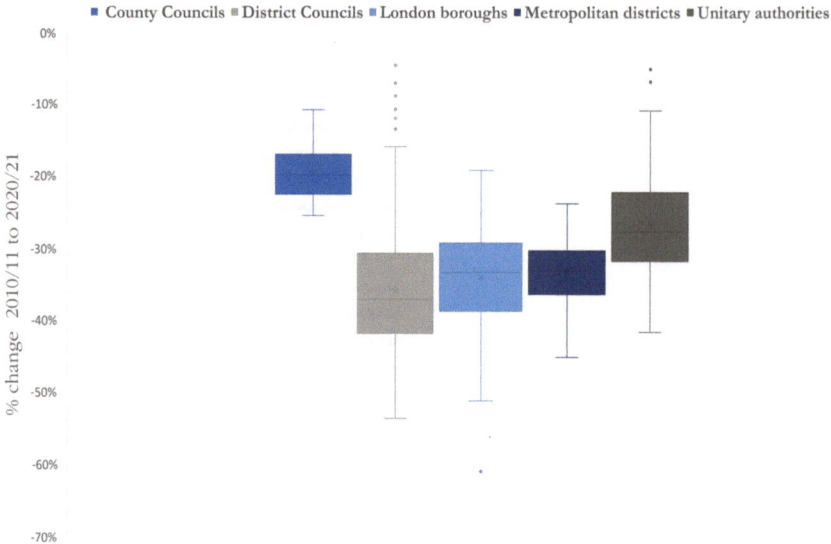

Fig. 5.3 Change in spending power per capita by local authority type in England 2010–2011 to 2020–2021 (stem and leaf plot showing range, IQ range and average). (*Source* Financial sustainability of local authorities visualisation: update—National Audit Office (NAO) report). nb average, range, and inter-quartile range shown

government involvement in the economy, and the instinctive preference to devolve increasing responsibility to the private sector and free market.

This aversion to government intervention in the economy can also be discerned in the UK's approach to industrial strategy over recent decades, with a shift away from the state-led economic planning and coordination, that was the norm through the mid-twentieth century, in favour of arms-length policies to promote greater competition and foreign direct investment (Arestis & Sawyer, 2005, 201–202). This shift has meant that key strategic industries have been starved of much-needed public investment, intervention, coordination, and support. Indeed, the lack of a clear state-led industrial strategy has been identified as an exacerbating factor in the relatively rapid decline of the UK's manufacturing sector, with adverse long-term effects on the resilience of the whole economy (Kitson & Michie, 2014). Again, this exemplifies the neoliberal belief that the roles and responsibilities of the state, particularly in relation to the economy,

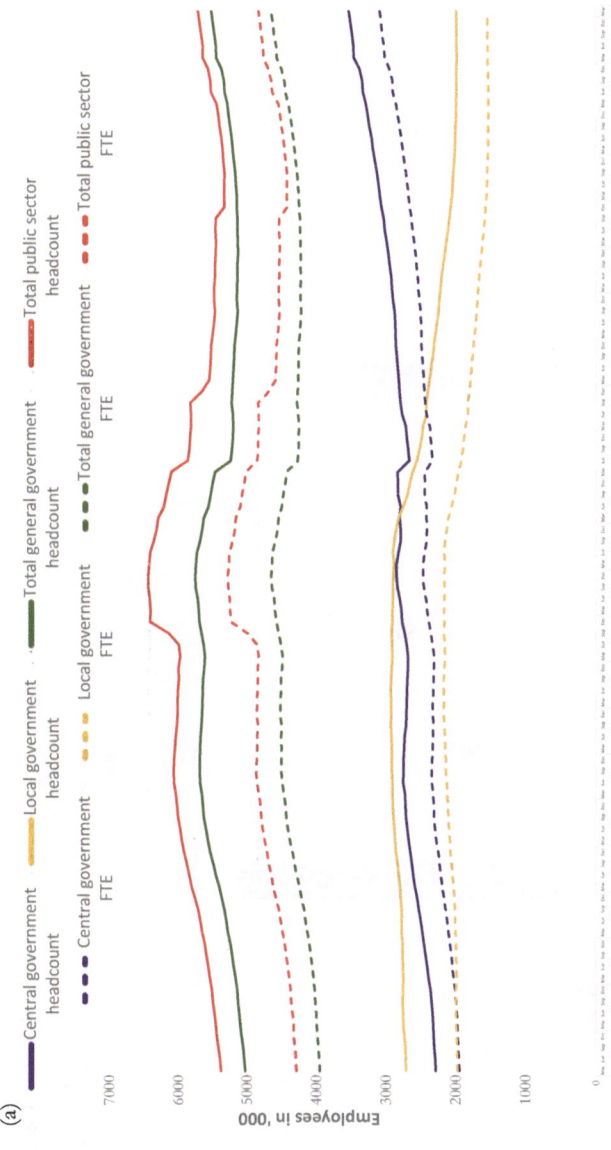

Fig. 5.4   a The UK state: Changes in state employment headcount and FTE ('000) (1999–2022), **b** Absolute and % changes in state employment by tier across the UK state 2008–2018 (*Source* Financial sustainability of local authorities visualisation: update—National Audit Office [NAO] report 2021)

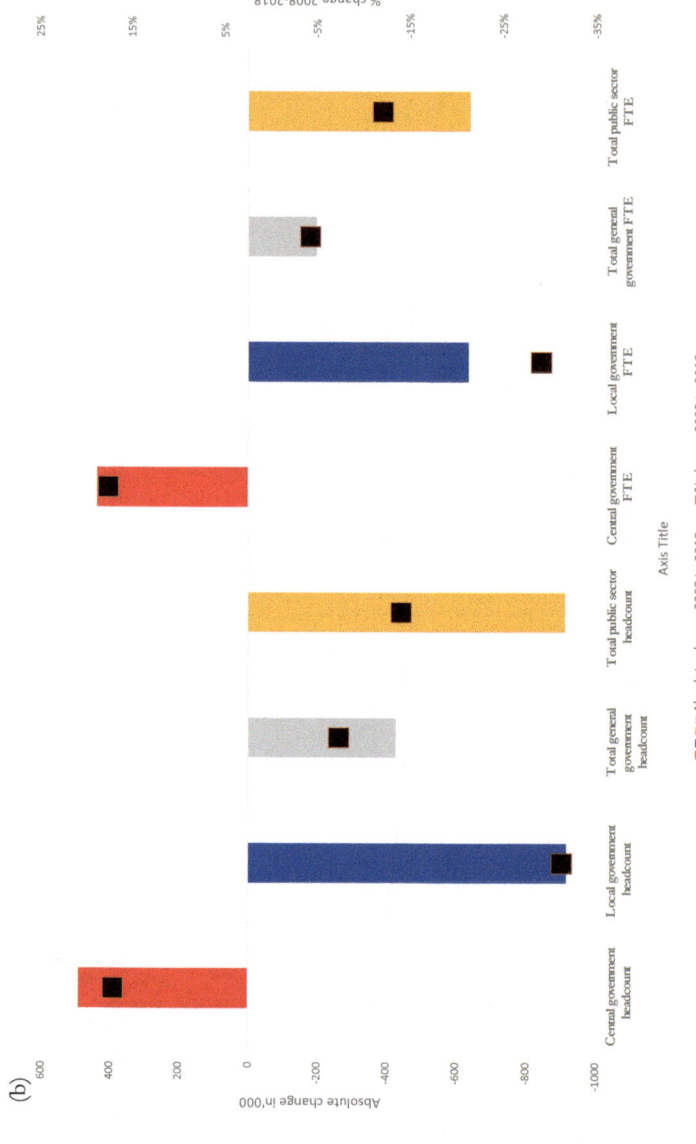

Fig. 5.4 (continued)

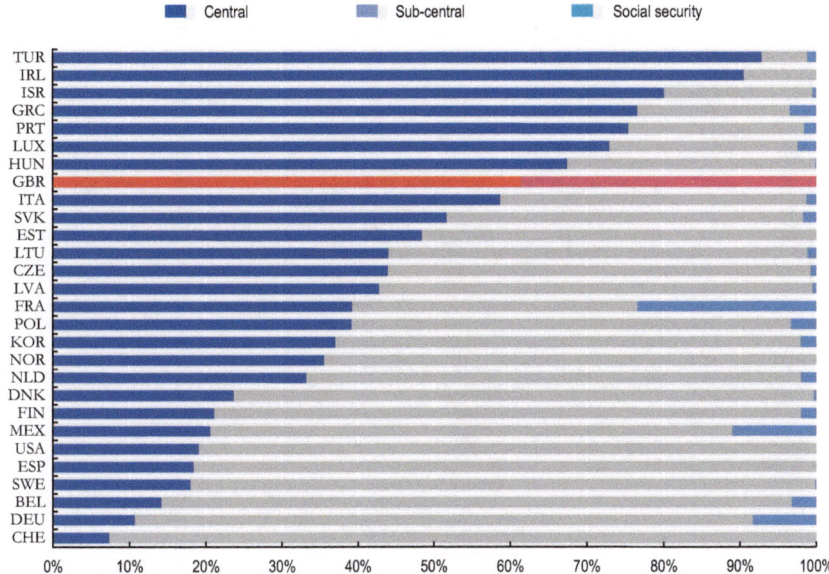

Fig. 5.5 Distribution of general government employment across levels of UK government in 2019 in OECD context (*Source* OECD Government at a glance, 2021)

should be minimised; that it is not the business of the state to seek to directly create jobs, support industries, or deliver services; that these aims can more efficiently and effectively be delivered by the free market.

Most recently, neoliberal logics about the roles and responsibilities of the state, and the idea that only a minimal state can be justified, have been actualised through the widespread and sustained austerity policies pursued by the UK government.

As noted above, cuts to local government funding, have eroded the capacity for many councils to effectively provide the vital front-line public services that communities rely upon (Gray & Barford, 2018, 541). Between 2010–2011 and 2017–2018, cuts to local government in England led to the closure of 500 children's centres and 340 libraries. Many councils' preventive housing services and local emergency welfare funds have also been decimated (UN, 2019).

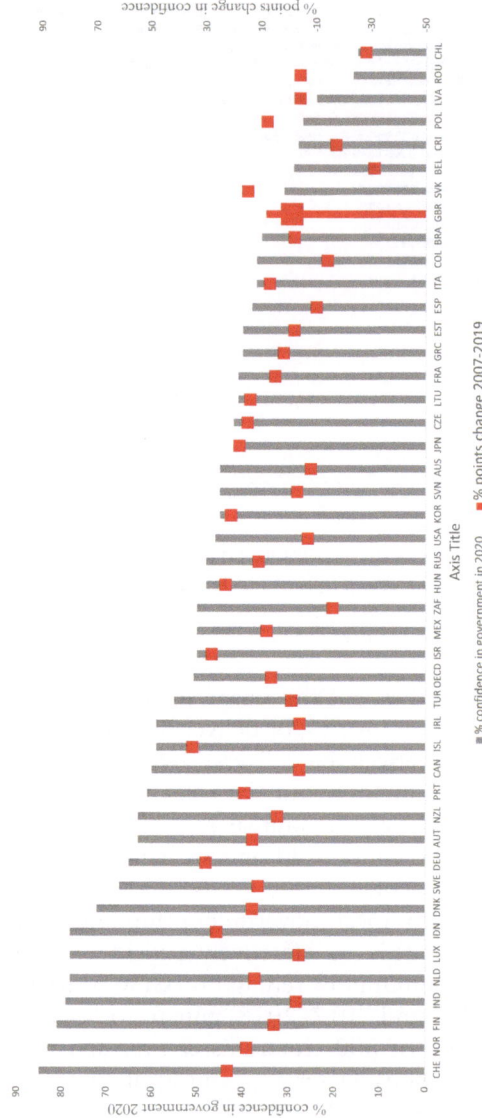

Fig. 5.6 Confidence in national government in 2020 and its change 2007–2020 (*Source* OECD Government at a glance, 2021)

Crucially, local public health budgets have not been immune to these cuts. The 'public health grant' paid to local authorities is 22 per cent lower in real terms in 2020/2021 than compared to 2015/2016 (The King's Fund, 2020). Analysis by the IPPR think tank has shown that the impacts of these cuts have fallen disproportionately on more deprived areas of the country, with the ten most deprived local authority areas in England bearing almost 15 per cent of all cuts and losing approximately 35p in every £1 of their public health budget (Thomas, 2019). These cuts have led to reductions in vital public health services, desperately needed to address widening health inequalities (Marmot et al., 2020), and have undermined local capacity to respond to health crises (Vize, 2020).

By steadily shrinking the roles, responsibilities, and resources of the state, at both a national and a local level, neoliberal policies of privatisation and public spending cuts, have left the British state both less willing, and less able, to act purposefully in an emergency situation such as the COVID-19 pandemic (Williams et al., 2021).

In such situations, states require the organisational capacity, resources, and institutional memory to respond effectively, dynamically, and decisively; expanding the roles and responsibilities of the state, at speed and scale, to meet public needs and protect public health. In this respect, East Asian states have been best in class. For example, South Korea was able to rapidly adopt a highly effective 'test, trace, isolate, and treat' system which was organised and managed in partnership between national and local governments. By expanding testing capacity in the early stages of the outbreak, the South Korean government was able to implement a strategy of early detection and containment of cases, with screening for travellers at the border, public testing stations, and mobile phone technologies adopted to support rapid testing and contact tracing (Majeed et al., 2020; Ministry of Health & Welfare, 2020).

In Taiwan, too, a proactive, state-led approach to pandemic control has enabled the country to avoid significant outbreaks of the virus. Like South Korea, Taiwan utilised information technology to support a real-time alert system, a precision testing strategy, and the effective surveillance of infected individuals in quarantine. Local government has also supported this system, with staff making daily phone calls to those under quarantine to offer assistance and provide care packages (Lee et al., 2020).

Such examples show the effectiveness of state-led coordination of public health measures, deploying the resources and organisational capacity of government to test, trace, and isolate cases of the virus at speed and scale, and helping to proactively halt the spread of the virus in the community.

In contrast to this international best practice, however, the UK government has, throughout the pandemic, instinctively sought market-based solutions to the COVID-19 crisis. For example, in England, contact tracing was initially carried out by Public Health England, working with local authorities. However, on 12th March 2020, as the number of cases in the community outstripped testing and tracing capacity, widespread contact tracing was stopped and resources reserved for those in hospitals and other high-risk settings. A new system, NHS Test and Trace, was launched on 28th May 2020 to increase national capacity. However, rather than using this system to rebuild local and regional public health capacity decimated by years of austerity, the UK Government instead created a complex web of public–private partnerships that utilises the NHS, Public Health England, university and military resources, as well as the services of private sector firms such as Deloitte, G4S, Serco, and Amazon. Despite costing £10 billion to establish, this system has faced significant challenges, shortcomings, and inefficiencies. For example, call handlers recruited by Serco were reportedly only able to trace around 60 per cent of contacts linked to the cases they are handling, hampering efforts to limit the spread of the virus (Briggs et al., 2020).

As it sought to scale-up testing capacity further, the UK government opted again for a public–private partnership model, overlooking the potential to expand existing public sector laboratory capacity, to establish a series of new 'lighthouse' mega laboratories across the country. However, unlike the existing NHS laboratory system, these lighthouse laboratories did not have the same level of supply chain management or logistical expertise, leading to unnecessary delays in returning test results (Williams et al., 2021, 218).

The outsourcing of large elements of the test and trace system to the private sector reflects the neoliberal prejudice against the state directly providing goods and services. Or, as the journalist Matthew D'Ancona (2020) puts it when describing the UK's approach to test and trace: "an almost religious belief that big private sector solutions are better than fragmented public services".

The Government's preference for, and reliance upon, the market during the pandemic can also be seen as a legacy of the UK's long-term deficit of clear, strategic industrial policy and relaxed attitude to the decline of strategic industries. The withering of domestic manufacturing capacity, and related supply chains, has left the UK exposed to endemic shortages of vital personal protective equipment (PPE) for health workers, ventilators, and other key medical supplies throughout the pandemic (Galloway, 2020; Saad-Filho, 2021, 135). Coupled with the Government's comparatively slow response to the pandemic, the UK's inability, let alone unwillingness, to commandeer significant domestic manufacturing capacity to produce health equipment meant the UK was left to fight for supplies on the global market amidst unprecedented demand. This led to farcical scenes, such as the shipment of PPE purchased for the NHS from Turkey which, once flown to the UK by the Royal Air Force and after much ministerial fanfare, was found to fall short of UK quality standards (Rawlinson, 2020).

Shortages of PPE in the early stages of a pandemic have been highlighted as a major factor responsible for the spread of COVID-19 in hospitals and care homes in England, leading to deaths amongst staff, patients and residents (McKee, 2020). These shortages may have also contributed to the UK's slow adoption of public mask-wearing as a way to limit infection. Indeed, concerns that public mask-wearing would threaten the supply of PPE to healthcare workers were highlighted by SAGE and meant the recommendation that the public wear a mask in public was delayed significantly (Fisher-Pearson & Mallet, 2020).

To reiterate, we do not mean to suggest here that the British state has not utilised its resources and capabilities whatsoever during the pandemic. Centralised planning, coordination, and redeployment of public sector capacity has played a critical role in the successful rollout of vaccines through the National Health Service. Similarly, the state has ramped up public spending to support businesses and individuals impacted by the pandemic, not least through the Coronavirus Job Retention Scheme (commonly known as 'furlough'), which helped to reduce potential redundancies across the labour market (Clark, 2021). Our point is that, at critical junctures throughout the pandemic, the UK government has demonstrated an unwillingness and inability to expand its roles and responsibilities in line with international best practice, instead showing an instinctive preference for, and reliance upon, the private sector and free market.

Again, this is not an accidental consequence of poor decision-making or incompetence by particular ministers or government officials. It is the predictable consequence, and continuation, of an ingrained neoliberal assumption, that the roles and responsibilities of the state should be minimised in favour of empowered and expanded markets. It is the predictable consequence too, of neoliberal policies that have, over recent decades, rolled back the state, eroded its resources, and depleted its capacity, leaving the state with neither the latitude nor the inclination for expansive and proactive intervention. Where the state and, its levers for action, have been steadily cut and diminished, the choice architecture available to policymakers in a crisis will be similarly limited, with fewer resources available to proactively control the situation. Meanwhile, it becomes harder to even consider utilising the full potential of the state in a crisis, let alone expanding its roles and responsibilities, without first overcoming significant cognitive dissonance. To do so requires pushing against the grain of received wisdom and assumptions about the possibility and probity of state intervention, entrenched over decades.

We can therefore see that the logics and legacies of neoliberalism have, again, hindered the UK government's response to the pandemic and unnecessarily threatened public health, promoting an approach to COVID-19 that has too often overlooked the potential of the state in favour of inefficient, and ineffective, private sector solutions that abdicate more and more responsibility for public welfare to the free market.

Towards a Republican State

This approach to thinking about the state, its roles and responsibilities is both politically contingent and unnecessary. As we saw in the previous chapter, the republican tradition of political thought offers a robust alternative to neoliberal ideas about freedom. It offers an equally robust alternative to neoliberal ideas about the state.

Recall that whilst neoliberals seem to hold that it is only possible to be free in a free market, with any potential for state interference and intervention minimised as far as possible, republicans hold that it is only possible to be free in a free state. It is the state that, through its legal and institutional architectures, neutralises the potential for powerful actors in society to wield arbitrary interference over others, guaranteeing each individual the intersubjective status of a free and equal citizen within that jurisdiction. On the republican view, therefore, it is not only legitimate and justifiable for the state to play a more active role in the economy and wider society, but desirable for the maintenance of freedom as non-domination (cf. Pettit, 1997, 148–150, 163). As Pettit states, so long as the state is constitutionally prevented from representing a source of discretionary power in its own right, republicans "will be well disposed towards a form of government that gives the law and the state a considerable range of responsibilities" (ibid., 150). Indeed, Pettit has explicitly challenged the neoliberal logic that only a minimal state can be justified, arguing that "[t]he state is not just to be a night watchman who protects against internal and external turmoil but an agency that moulds and shapes society" (2010, 39).

The distinction between arbitrary and non-arbitrary interference enables republicans to adopt a more optimistic, and expansive account of the state, its roles, and responsibilities. It is entirely permissible for the state to intervene in the market, deliver public services, or, indeed, own and operate economic enterprises (O'Shea, 2020; Pettit, 1996, 590–592; 1997, 158–163), in so far as these actions are pursued in the public interest, and are legally and constitutionally governed to ensure they cannot, in and of themselves, represent a form of dominating arbitrary interference. This includes pursuing policies to support high levels of employment, to develop domestic industrial and commercial capacity, and to invest in the maintenance of a functioning welfare state (Pettit, 1997, 158–165).

The republican argument in favour of an expansive, rather than minimal, the state is further strengthened by the extent to which state-led institutions and public services are not just compatible with citizens' freedom as non-domination, but critical to advancing this freedom. An expansive republican state can, through its various activities, provide individuals with the material and institutional bases for personal independence, empowering them against potential sources of domination that may arise in society (cf. Pettit, 1996, 590–592; 1997, 158–160). There are reasons to think that public health systems are a paradigmatic example of the way that states, acting in the common interest, can help to reinforce citizens' defences against domination in their lives. By providing effective healthcare to the public, the state is able to protect citizens from dependency on the exploitative, discretionary power of private healthcare providers to choose who to treat, and how much to charge them (ibid.).

From the republican view, then, there is no need to instinctively prefer, or rely upon, private sector solutions to public challenges. Nor would there be a need to pursue a policy agenda that seeks to continually shrink the state, its roles, and responsibilities as much as possible. Faced with a global pandemic, this republican understanding of the state and its potential would have enabled a more enthusiastic and proactive state-led response in the UK, one that would have been more in line with the international best-practice exemplified in South Korea and Taiwan. Had the resources and capacities of the British state not been unnecessarily diminished over recent decades in pursuit of some ideal, minimal state, there would have been greater opportunity to commandeer and redeploy public assets to support the public health effort, and avoid the delay and dysfunctionality in the private sector that has cost lives. In other words, promoting a republican account of the state could have helped to increase both the willingness and the ability of the UK government to intervene proactively in the common interests of public health and public welfare throughout the pandemic, utilising the full capacity of the public sector to effectively test, trace, isolate, and treat COVID-19 and limit it's spread in the community. Only by challenging neoliberal assumptions about the roles and responsibilities of the state, and reversing the damage inflicted by decades of rampant privatisation, negligent industrial strategy, and fiscal austerity, can we hope to rebuild the UK's resilience, and its capacity to respond to crises in the public interest.

Conclusion

In his book, *Late Victorian Holocausts*, Mike Davis (2002) documented the unprecedented human suffering which has been visited on the poor historically by dint of the reticence of some governments to interfere in the machinations of markets. This argument cannot be applied easily or simply or perhaps even at all to the UK's government's neoliberal-informed response to the pandemic. As a disaster event COVID-19 cannot be compared to the El Niño-Southern Oscillation-related famines of 1876–1878, 1896–1897 and 1899–1902 in India, China, Brazil, Ethiopia, Korea, Vietnam, the Philippines, and New Caledonia that Davis examines. Furthermore, nineteenth-century Malthusian laissez-faire economics clearly differs in important ways from twenty-first-century market fundamentalism. Still, there is something in Davis' account that haunts the neoliberal present; to suppose that state intervention is essentially unhelpful—and perhaps even immoral—is to prepare to fail, with life and death consequences. It is to enter a pandemic event with a cognitive disability that makes it doubly more difficult to do what needs to be done.

REFERENCES

Arestis, P., & Sawyer, M. (2005). The neoliberal experience in the United Kingdom. In A. Saad-Filho & D. Johnston (Eds.), *Neoliberalism: A critical reader* (pp. 199–207). Pluto Press.

Berry, C. (2019). From receding to reseeding: Industrial policy, governance strategies and neoliberal resilience in post-crisis Britain. *New Political Economy, 25*(4), 607–625.

Briggs, A., et al. (2020). NHS test and trace: The journey so far. https://www.health.org.uk/publications/long-reads/nhs-test-and-trace-the-journey-so-far. Accessed 28 Dec 2021.

Clark, H. (2021). Examining the end of the furlough scheme. https://commonslibrary.parliament.uk/examining-the-end-of-the-furlough-scheme/. Accessed 28 Dec 2021.

D'Ancona, M. (2020) Hancock is GREAT. https://members.tortoisemedia.com/2020/10/05/201005-test-and-trace-slow-news-audio-hancock-is-great-plus-transcript/content.html. Accessed 28 Dec 2021.

Davies, M. (2002). *Late Victorian Holocausts: El Niño Famines and the Making of the Third World*. Verso.

Fisher-Pearson, N., & Mallet, J. (2020). Unmasking the failings: Why the UK government was too slow on face coverings. https://cherwell.org/2020/08/09/unmasking-the-failings-why-the-uk-government-was-too-slow-on-face-coverings/. Accessed 28 Dec 2021.

Galloway, L. (2020). Building a domestic manufacturing capacity. http://www.pharmatimes.com/web_exclusives/Building_a_domestic_manufacturing_capacity_1341929. Accessed 28 Dec 2021.

Gray, M., & Barford, A. (2018). The depths of the cuts: The uneven geography of local government austerity. *Cambridge Journal of Regions, Economy and Society, 11*(3), 541–563.

Hall, S. (2011). The neoliberal revolution. *Soundings, 48*, 9–27.

Harvey, D. (2005). *A brief history of neoliberalism*. Oxford University Press.

Johns, M. (2020). 10 years of austerity: Eroding resilience in the north. https://www.ippr.org/files/2020-06/10-years-of-austerity.pdf. Accessed 16 Dec 2021.

Kitson, M., & Michie, J. (2014). *The deindustrial revolution: The rise and fall of UK manufacturing, 1870–2010* (Centre for Business Research, University of Cambridge Working Paper, 459), pp. 1–38.

Lee, P., et al. (2020). What we can learn from Taiwan's response to the COVID-19 epidemic. https://blogs.bmj.com/bmj/2020/07/21/what-we-can-learn-from-taiwans-response-to-the-covid-19-epidemic/. Accessed 28 Dec 2021.

Majeed, A., et al. (2020). Can the UK emulate the South Korean approach to COVID-19? https://www.bmj.com/content/369/bmj.m2084 Accessed 28 Dec 2021.

Marmot, M., et al. (2020). *Health equity in England: The Marmot review 10 years on*. Institute of Health Equity.

McKee, M. (2020). England's PPE procurement failures must never happen again. https://www.bmj.com/content/370/bmj.m2858. Accessed 28 Dec 2021.

Ministry of Health and Welfare. (2020). COVID-19 response. http://ncov. mohw.go.kr/en/baroView.do?brdId=11&brdGubun=111&dataGubun=&ncvContSeq=&contSeq=&board_id=. Accessed 28 Dec 2021.

Mudge, S. L. (2008). What is neo-liberalism? *Socio-Economic Review, 6*, 703–731.

Munck, R. (2005). Neoliberalism and politics, and the politics of neoliberalism. In A. Saad-Filho & D. Johnston (Eds.), *Neoliberalism: A critical reader* (pp. 60–69). Pluto Press.

National Audit Office [NAO]. (2013). The role of major contractors in the delivery of public services. https://www.nao.org.uk/wp-content/uploads/2013/11/10296-001-Delivery-of-public-services-HC-8101.pdf. Accessed 28 Dec 2021.

Nozick, R. (1974). *Anarchy, state, and utopia*. Blackwell.

Organisation for Economic Co-operation and Development [OECD]. (2021). *Government at a glance*. OECD.

O'Shea, T. (2020). In defence of public ownership: A reply to Frye. *Political Theory, 48*(5), 581–587.

Pettit, P. (1996). Freedom as anti-power. *Ethics, 106*(3), 576–604.

Pettit, P. (1997). *Republicanism: A theory of freedom and government*. Oxford University Press.

Pettit, P. (2010). Civic republican theory. In J. L. Martí & P. Pettit (Eds.), *A political philosophy in public life: Civic republicanism in Zapatero's Spain*. Princeton University Press.

Rawlinson, K. (2020). Coronavirus PPE: All 400,000 gowns flown from Turkey for NHS fail UK standards. https://www.theguardian.com/world/2020/may/07/all-400000-gowns-flown-from-turkey-for-nhs-fail-uk-standards. Accessed 28 Dec 2021.

Rhodes, C., Hough, D., & Butcher, L. (2014). *Privatisation* (House of Commons Library Research Paper No. 14/61). House of Commons Library.

Saad-Filho, A. (2021). Endgame: From crisis in neoliberalism to crises of neoliberalism. *Human Geography, 14*(1), 133–137.

The King's Fund. (2020). Public health: Our position. https://www.kingsfund.org.uk/projects/positions/public-health. Accessed 28 Dec 2021.

Thomas, C. (2019). *Hitting the poorest worst? How public health cuts have been experienced in England's most deprived communities*. https://www.ippr.org/blog/public-health-cuts. Accessed 9 Nov 2022.

United Nations [UN]. (2019). Visit to the United Kingdom of Great Britain and Northern Ireland: Report of the special rapporteur on extreme poverty and human rights. https://undocs.org/A/HRC/41/39/Add.1. Accessed 28 Dec 2020.

Vallier, K. (2021). *Neoliberalism.* https://plato.stanford.edu/archives/sum 2021/entries/neoliberalism/. Accessed 28 Dec 2021.

Vize, R. (2020). How the erosion of our public health system hobbled England's COVID-19 response. https://www.bmj.com/content/369/bmj.m1934. Accessed 28 Dec 2021.

Williams, G. A., Rajan, R., & Cylus, J. D. (2021). COVID-19 in the United Kingdom: How austerity and a loss of state capacity undermined the crisis response. In S. L. Greer, E. J. King, E. M. da Fonseca, & A. Peralta-Santos (Eds.), *Coronavirus politics: The comparative politics and policy of COVID-19* (pp. 215–234). University of Michigan Press.

World Health Organisation [WHO]. (2020, March 5). WHO Director-General's opening remarks at the media briefing on COVID-19. https://www.who.int/director-general/speeches/detail/who-director-general-s-opening-rem arks-at-the-media-briefing-on-covid-19---5-march-2020. Accessed 5 May 2022.

CHAPTER 6

Me, Myself, and I? The Neoliberal Citizen

Abstract Neoliberal theory considers the market to be the primary space in which individuals can meaningfully exercise their agency, realise their freedom, and pursue their interests. This normative assumption has consequences for the role, responsibility, and power of the citizen, and the model of democratic politics promoted by neoliberals; expecting citizens to accept more and more personal risk and responsibility, whilst simultaneously undermining their capacity to wield control over their lives through the democratic state. This neoliberal vision of citizenship helps to explain why the UK state has repeatedly emphasised the personal, rather than collective, responsibility of citizens during the COVID-19 pandemic, whilst at the same time offering limited democratic oversight of the decisions and actions taken by government during the crisis. In this respect, the UK response can be understood as a continuation of pre-existing trends towards the corrosion of democratic citizenship, with efforts to 'depoliticise' policymaking decisions, and cultivate ideal neoliberal subjects that express their interests first and foremost through market choices rather than political participation.

Keywords Citizenship · Libertarianism · Freedom as non-interference · Democratic deficit · Post-politics · Sovereign political subject · Public square

M. Boyle et al., *COVID-19 and the Case Against Neoliberalism*, https://doi.org/10.1007/978-3-031-18935-7_6

INTRODUCTION

As we have seen throughout this book, neoliberal theory considers the market to be the primary space in which individuals can meaningfully exercise their agency, realise their freedom, and pursue their interests. This normative assumption has consequences for the role, responsibility, and power of the citizen in the model of democratic politics promoted by neoliberals; expecting citizens to accept more and more personal risk and responsibility, whilst simultaneously undermining their capacity to wield control over their lives through the democratic state.

This particular, neoliberal vision of citizenship helps to explain why the UK state has repeatedly emphasised the personal, rather than collective, responsibility of citizens during the COVID-19 pandemic, whilst at the same time offering limited democratic oversight of the decisions and actions taken by the government during the crisis. This stance towards UK citizens has left many exposed to impossible risk beyond their control, especially those who had no other choice but to continue working, often without adequate protection, in the face of a deadly pandemic. In this respect, the UK response can be understood as a continuation of pre-existing trends towards the corrosion of democratic citizenship, with efforts to 'depoliticise' policymaking decisions, and cultivate ideal neoliberal subjects that express their interests first and foremost through market choices rather than political participation.

DENUDED CITIZENSHIP AND THE CULTIVATION OF NEOLIBERAL SUBJECTS

Neoliberal theory is grounded on a normative ideal of the individual as a sovereign economic agent, able to act according to their own ideas and interests without facing patronising, paternalistic, or otherwise inhibiting interference from others, not least the state. Individuals ought therefore to be entrepreneurial and self-reliant, taking personal responsibility for their own lives (Brown, 2005, 42; Harvey, 2005, 23; Thorsen, 2010, 203). In order to cultivate such ideal neoliberal subjects, the state should withhold from interfering in the way individuals choose to live their lives. This includes forms of support or insurance that could prevent individuals from taking responsibility for their own actions and decisions, with the concept of the welfare state, in particular, cast by neoliberals as "the arch enemy of freedom" (Hall, 2011, 10).

This animosity towards welfare states is reflected, too, in the libertarian-leaning political theory of John Tomasi, who argues there is "a special form of self-esteem that comes when people recognize themselves as central causes of the particular lives they are living – rather than being in any way the ward of others, no matter how well meaning, other-regarding, or wise those others might be" (2012, 61). For Tomasi, welfare states and other forms of social safety net, by incubating people from risk and the need to plan financially for negative eventualities (such as poor health or unemployment) themselves, represent "a gilded cage" that prevents individuals from being able to direct their own lives (ibid., 113). As Tomasi explains, "A society that denies people the chance to take up questions of long-term financial planning for themselves, or that restricts the ways in which individuals and families can respond to such questions, thereby diminishes the capacity of citizens to become fully responsible and independent agents" (ibid., 80–81).

However, this reification of personal responsibility, and the abdication of collective responsibility—via the state—for the welfare of all citizens, means that the burdens and risks of social life become individualised and personalised. Expected to live by their own skill, luck, and competitive advantages, with limited social insurance for those who, by chance or happenstance, are disadvantaged by the function and outcomes of the free market, the promotion of personal responsibility by neoliberals is, in effect, a promotion of intense precarity for many citizens (Näsström & Kalm, 2015). Exposed to the possibilities of hunger, destitution, and poverty for themselves and their families, neoliberal citizens bear the responsibility, and the consequences, of failure to faultlessly navigate the vagaries and exigencies of an increasingly marketised society. With few protections available, this neoliberal 'precariat' are perpetually vulnerable, "knowing that one mistake or one piece of bad luck could tip the balance" (Standing, 2011, 20). Meanwhile the possibility of easing this vulnerability through the collective maintenance of a shared social safety net—below which nobody may fall, regardless of their ability to compete successfully in the market—is considered by neoliberals to be incompatible with individual liberty.

Indeed, for theorists such as Tomasi, this individualised risk and precarity is not just an acceptable consequence of market competition, it is a positively desirable one. The experience of risk, Thomasi argues, is "an essential precondition for...self-respect". Welfare systems that "insulate people from economic risks" deny them "opportunities to feel the special sense that they have done something genuinely important with their lives" (2012, 80). Paradoxically, perhaps, it is only through exposure to the uncontrollable consequences of failure in a competitive market, then, that individuals can experience the agency and autonomy of sovereign economic agents, and feel in control of their own lives.

The legacies of this reification of personal responsibility within actually existing neoliberal policymaking are clearly discernible. Over recent decades, there has been a "great risk shift" (Hacker, 2006), with the transfer of economic risk away from institutions of social insurance (previously established by the state, employers, and communities) and onto the shoulders of individual citizens. In the UK, the steady erosion of the post-1945 welfare state, and with it the idea of social insurance against shared risks, has accelerated with the introduction of austerity policies. For example, spending on non-pensioner benefits has been falling since 2012/2013; and since 2016 a 'benefits freeze' has meant that these no longer keep up with inflation (Joseph Rowntree Foundation, 2020, 51), leaving many benefit claimants unable to make ends meet. As the benefits system has been made less generous and less effective at protecting those most in need from poverty, it has been made more conditional, with punitive sanctions regimes introduced (Wright et al., 2020). Missing just one Jobcentre appointment can now see benefit payments reduced or removed completely for 28 days. Indeed, almost a quarter of all jobseeker's allowance claimants were sanctioned between 2010 and 2015 (NAO, 2016). The net effect of this has been to transform the welfare state from a valued foundation of collective insurance to a poverty trap—designed less to provide people with a right to help when they need it most and more to dissuade people from the idea that the state should (or can) help at all.

The neoliberal retreat from the idea that the welfare of people and communities lies within the purview of the democratic state—that, indeed, ensuring the economy functions effectively for all people and places is one of the great opportunities of democracy—has been accompanied by a devaluation of democracy, and democratic citizenship, more broadly. When market relations come to take such a central normative role in human life, the value and importance of democratic participation are diminished. If it is the market where we exercise our freedom, express our agency, and generate social good, what need do we have for expansive democratic politics?

As Harvey notes, neoliberals are "profoundly suspicious of democracy" (2005, 66), concerned that the whims of the democratic public could unduly influence or upset the function and outcomes of free market exchange. As a result, neoliberalism tends towards depoliticisation and technocratic governance, as well as an 'economization' (Brown, 2015, 17) of those elements of democratic politics that remain. This is not to suggest that neoliberals are necessarily antidemocratic; representative democracy is, after all, often considered by neoliberals to be instrumentally valuable as an effective model of legislative governance and as a check on tyranny (Vallier, 2021). But democratic engagement by ordinary citizens is not seen as something that is inherently valuable, nor should it be deepened, strengthened, and expanded. Instead, democracy should be limited, downplayed, and "devalorised" (Munck, 2005, 66), with the quotidian business of politics abdicated to professional politicians, technocrats, and 'apolitical' experts.

This attempt to insulate governance from the influence of democratic 'politics', with appeals to apolitical expertise, efficiency, and pragmatism, is itself inherently political. Not only does it have implications for the location of power in society (via the disempowerment of ordinary citizens), but it also informs the 'Overton window' of acceptable policymaking. Neoliberal technocrats stick to the script of neoliberal policymaking, implementing neoliberal agendas and perpetuating neoliberal assumptions about what is possible and permissible (Gallo, 2021, 5). This is what gives rise to a sense of (neoliberal) capitalist realism: 'There Is No Alternative', and there are few avenues for citizens to demand, design, and deliver one through a professionalised representative politics.

In particular, by seeking to protect the function and outcomes of the market from political influence (Mudge, 2008, 715), neoliberals extinguish the potential for meaningful democratic control over the economy. Indeed, neoliberals hold that citizens can more effectively and efficiently express their ideas and interests as market actors than political ones. As the sociologist Ronaldo Munck argues: "[t]he complex and empowering vision of citizenship in its classic democratic presentation was reduced, in the era of neoliberalism, to the power of the credit card and the pleasures of the shopping mall" (2005, 65)]. The neoliberal model therefore promotes a denuded public sphere, and an infantilised democracy—one in which citizens are not understood to be equal, active participants in the political life of their communities, but instead merely political-consumers who (infrequently) have the opportunity to vote for electoral candidates.

By reifying the logics, processes, and outcomes of the market, neoliberalism "assaults the principles, practices, cultures, subjects, and institutions of democracy understood as rule by the people" (Brown, 2015, 9). Under neoliberalism, the state is not a democratically co-owned and cooperated enterprise for actively discovering and pursuing the common good, but merely a tolerated guarantor of market functions. And as such, under the neoliberal state, the future is not to be shaped politically by the needs, aspirations, and imaginations of democratic citizens, but by the aggregated economic outcomes of free market exchange.

The legacies of this neoliberal suspicion of democracy and preference for depoliticisation can be revealed in the recent political history of the UK. The political scientist Peter Burnham, for example, has identified depoliticisation as "a distinctive form of statecraft" deployed by the Blair government, *"placing at one remove the political character of decision-making"* (2001, 128 emphasis in original). By embracing technocratic governance, and shifting power away from governing politicians to external organisations, bodies, and agencies, the Blair government could deny responsibility for "the consequences of unpopular policies" whilst also increasing its credibility with financial markets (ibid., 129). A key example of this depoliticisation can be seen in the introduction of 'operational independence' in the area of monetary policy to the Bank of England in 1997. Passing the responsibility for setting interest rates to the independent Bank of England allowed New Labour to seemingly elevate monetary policy above politics, insulating it from democratic interference whilst also shielding the government from any public dissatisfaction with high-interest rates and currency inflation (ibid., 137–139). As with the large-scale privatisation of public assets, nationalised industries, and state-run firms, the 'depoliticisation' of monetary policy can be understood as an attempt to place the market beyond the control of democratic citizens. Citizens can no longer hold democratic governments properly accountable for great swathes of economic policy that have been left to the cold calculations of both market processes or economic technocrats. The power of the democratic state has been curtailed, and the influence of the democratic citizen minimised. There Is No Alternative.

The suspicion of democracy contained within such neoliberal policymaking, and the emphasis on transactional, technocratic forms of governance rather than the democratic self-rule of an empowered citizenry, has coincided with a broader weakening of civic engagement in the UK. Despite some modest improvements in recent years, turnout in elections, voter registration, and membership of political parties and trade unions all remain well below mid-twentieth century levels; with the sharpest declines in these forms of political participation occurring with the arrival of neoliberal hegemony in the 1980s (Audickas et al., 2019; Department for Business, Energy & Industrial Strategy, 2020; James, 2018). Why value participation in democratic politics, when the state is presented as impotent in the face of market economics?

The model of neoliberal citizenship presented here, then, can be categorised as one of responsibility without power. Citizens are expected to individually shoulder (indeed, embrace!) the risks and uncertainties of market competition, whilst abdicating the power to control these risks and uncertainties through the collective command of the democratic state. Citizenship is about accepting personal responsibility for our own lives, rather than exercising collective responsibility for the lives of our community as democratic citizens.

Throughout the COVID-19 pandemic, this neoliberal responsibility-without-power conception of citizenship can be seen to have underpinned the UK government's approach; a reflexive instinct that policymakers have returned to repeatedly throughout the crisis. In the absence of pre-emptive state intervention and consistent guidance, individual citizens have been expected to accept significant personal responsibility for navigating the social challenge presented by the pandemic, weighing the personal risk of infection against the need to keep working and socialising. Yet, simultaneously, they have had few formal avenues through which to democratically engage with, scrutinise, and influence, the government policy- and decision-making that impacts their capacity to tackle the social challenge of COVID-19.

Any pandemic is, inherently, a collective action problem. Pandemics are a consequence of human beings' social nature; of our lives lived together in families, schools, workplaces, and communities. And as such, they are a question of how, together, human beings can best fight the spread of infection, protect public health, wellbeing and prosperity, and prevent unnecessary harm befalling each other. Certainly, we all have a personal responsibility to do what we can to protect the safety of others in such circumstances, but to be effective, our individual responses to the pandemic need to be organised and coordinated collectively. Atomised individuals cannot fight a pandemic alone.

Nevertheless, the UK government has repeatedly chosen to emphasise individual personal responsibility as the key to fighting COVID-19.

This can be seen, for example, in the shift in government messaging in May 2020 from the clear directive to "Stay home, protect the NHS, save lives" to the more ambiguous "Stay alert, control the virus, save lives" (Evans, 2021). This new request that the public 'stay alert' was introduced precisely as the government began to lift the first national lockdown that had been imposed two months earlier, implying that it was now the responsibility of individuals to prevent further waves of infection even as the government was implicitly and explicitly encouraging the public to return to work, and resume socialising in shops, pubs, and restaurants whilst the risk from the virus remained high.

This emphasis on personal responsibility was put even more bluntly by the Prime Minister, Boris Johnson, in December 2020. The second national lockdown had ended on 2nd December, yet cases were still rising rapidly. With the government reluctant to impose restrictions in the run-up to Christmas, despite the increased risk of transmission created by festive socialising, the Prime Minister deflected responsibility on to the public: "this Christmas it's vital that everyone exercises the greatest possible personal responsibility" (Johnson, 2020). Rather than setting clear, shared rules and guidelines to prevent transmission rates spiralling further out of control, the Prime Minister suggested that individuals "think hard and in detail about the days ahead and whether you can do more to protect yourself and others".

Asking individuals to take such personal responsibility for the pandemic may be fine in theory, but this underappreciates the limitations many people may face in pursuing the collective interests of public health in their day-to-day life. These limitations may be due to a lack of personal knowledge about the virus and how it spreads, but may also be due to economic and social factors; not least the need to continue working, return to school, or care for loved ones.

This is only exacerbated in the absence of a sufficient safety net to support those who are disproportionately impacted by the pandemic. For example, at £95.85 a week, the UK has one of the lowest rates of minimum statutory sick pay in Europe, and almost 2 million employees are not eligible for sick pay at all. This has meant that many individuals have felt unable to self-isolate when exposed to COVID-19 or when sick themselves, with an impossible choice between the responsibility to protect public health and the need to make ends meet (TUC, 2021). In such a context, the government calls for personal responsibility suggest both an acceptance of the state's unwillingness and/or inability to protect citizens on a collective basis, and a nonchalance about the unequal mortal threat faced by certain members of society who may be more exposed to the risk of infection as a result of the economic necessity to continue going out to work during a pandemic (rather than working from home or drawing an income from other sources, such as rent).

Again, we do not mean to suggest that the government has abdicated responsibility for the pandemic entirely. The introduction of lockdown measures, as well as support packages for businesses and individuals impacted by the restrictions, have shown that coordinated collective action has still been the primary state response to the pandemic, even where these interventions have been hesitant, reluctant, or piecemeal. Our more nuanced claim, instead, is that the UK government has repeatedly and reflexively acquiesced to a particular neoliberal instinct, reifying personal responsibility. This, in turn, has limited the efficacy of the overall state response to COVID-19 at critical junctures.

The repeated emphasis on personal responsibility seen in the UK during the pandemic appears to go against the grain of much international best practice. For example, in New Zealand the government has adopted clear and consistent messaging throughout the pandemic, stressing the collective, solidaristic effort required to curb infections. Citizens were described as a "Team of 5 million" who needed to "Unite against COVID-19" (Exeter et al., 2020, 5). Such language contrasts markedly with the UK government's neoliberal delegation of responsibility to individuals and reflects the reality that any effective response to a pandemic will necessarily be collective in nature.

Meanwhile, the neoliberal instinct to depoliticise, and elevate areas of policy beyond the purview of democratic scrutiny, can also be seen to have shaped the UK government's response to COVID-19. The government have repeatedly sought to limit debate around their pandemic policies, insisting these have been "guided by the science" rather than political ideas, intuitions, or judgements (Kettell & Kerr, 2022). By drawing on the status, reliability, and neutrality associated with medical and scientific expertise, such a narrative allowed the government to present their decisions as "out of their hands" (ibid., 15). This enabled the government to shut down consideration of possible alternatives whilst simultaneously limiting their potential exposure to any criticisms of their chosen course of action (ibid.). Such depoliticisation, however, reduces the opportunity for citizens to adequately engage in, and scrutinise, political decision-making during the pandemic.

It is vital that robust scientific knowledge, intelligence, and expertise are available to inform policymaking. But by emphasising the role of SAGE and other scientific advisers in determining policy, there is an implicit signal from the government to the public that there is no other possible course of action that the government could possibly take, and no possibility to reconsider this approach in the light of public ideas, needs, or interests.

An aversion to democratic scrutiny can also be seen in the government's repeated reliance on emergency powers, bringing new public health measures into force before these had been deliberated and approved by Members of Parliament (MPs). Indeed, the preference of the government was often to announce such restrictions via managed briefings to the media (or even leaks to favoured journalists), rather than parliamentary debates (Nice, 2020). With democratic representatives marginalised, any democratic scrutiny by citizens themselves appeared to be largely tokenistic, for example, with the introduction of pre-recorded questions from members of the public during televised government press briefings. Meanwhile, the independent public inquiry into the government's handling of the pandemic would not commence until 2022, with Boris Johnson arguing that it was necessary to avoid adding pressure on the government, its advisers, and the NHS while the risk from the virus remained high (*BBC News*, 2021). This delay to the inquiry process meant that citizens lost yet another opportunity to scrutinise public decision-making, and shape its course, while the pandemic was still unfolding.

Elsewhere, however, democratic engagement and scrutiny have been more valued. For example, in January 2021 the Scottish Parliament convened a citizens' panel to discuss the question: 'What priorities should shape the Scottish Government's approach to COVID-19 restrictions and strategy in 2021?'. Over four weekends, the panel took evidence from a range of scientific and medical experts, scrutinised the Scottish Government's approach to the pandemic so far, and considered which priorities should inform this approach in future. The findings were then reported to the Scottish Parliament's Covid-19 Committee, ensuring that the ideas and interests of a representative sample of Scottish citizens could inform the future approach to fighting COVID-19 in Scotland (The Scottish Parliament, 2021). Whilst hardly revolutionary, such democratic engagement appears in stark contrast with the minimalistic, tokenistic, and technocratic approach to policy- and decision-making adopted by the UK government in Westminster. Indeed, paradoxically, the UK government appears to have instead adopted precisely the cliched model of patronising, distant, and ineffective state bureaucracy that neoliberalism purports to reject.

Throughout the pandemic, then, the UK government has reflected neoliberal assumptions about the role and value of citizens in a democracy, displaying these instincts through its emphasis on personal responsibility, and its devaluation of democratic scrutiny. Again, this highlights the political contingency of the UK government's approach which, far from representing the outcome of discrete decisions by particular policymakers, can be understood as a continuation of broader neoliberal trends and commitments in UK policymaking over recent decades.

The Republican Conception
of the Vigilant Citizen

This neoliberal approach adopted towards citizens, citizenship, and the idea of democracy more broadly, during the pandemic was not inevitable or necessary. And once again, the republican tradition of political thought offers an available alternative that policymakers have overlooked.

From a republican perspective, the neoliberal emphasis on personal responsibility as a normative value appears, at best, short-sighted and; at worst, a threat to liberty. Recall that, for republicans, the state has the potential to represent a machine through which citizens can promote their common welfare—that is, their shared interest in freedom as non-domination. As Pettit states, the aim of a republican state should be "to do all it can to increase the intensity with which people enjoy non-domination" (1997, 106). As we have already seen, reducing the sources of domination faced by individuals in society requires the state to maintain expansive protective, regulatory, and empowering institutions (such as public health and education systems) that function to neutralise the capacity of powerful agents to wield arbitrary interference in the lives of their fellow citizens (Pettit, 1996, 589–592; 1997, 158–160).

Both republicans and neoliberals seek to promote personal independence. But whilst neoliberals see this as requiring individuals to be self-reliant and to take full responsibility for their own lives, republicans see personal independence as politically and institutionally constituted in common; guaranteed through the state, not despite it. It is therefore unlikely that a suitably republican state would abdicate responsibility for a collective challenge like a global pandemic to individual citizens. Doing so could risk the freedom of citizens as they fall vulnerable to exploitation or manipulation by others, for example, being compelled to return to work despite the risks this could pose to public health.

The promotion of republican liberty therefore requires a more solidaristic and communitarian (cf. Pettit, 1997, 120–126) conception of citizenship than that promoted by neoliberals: republican citizens are not atomised individuals responsible only for promoting their own self-interest, they instead have a common interest in the collective promotion of freedom as non-domination through the maintenance of a republican state (and its associated public welfare institutions) in concert with their fellow citizens. Indeed, it is only through the maintenance of such a state that individuals are able to enjoy the intersubjective status of free and equal republican citizenship with others in their community. This republican account of citizenship aligns much more closely with the approach taken in New Zealand where fighting the pandemic has consistently been framed as a collective effort, than the UK where fighting the pandemic has repeatedly been framed as a personal responsibility of individuals.

But more than this, from a republican perspective, the capacity of the state to abdicate responsibility for a collective challenge—a threat to the common welfare of all citizens—would represent a form of discretionary, dominating power in its own right. Indeed, a government that, through carelessness or contempt, can allow thousands of citizens to bear unnecessary risk and harm would represent a distinct threat to liberty. Such a government would hold the capacity to act arbitrarily, with no constitutional or democratic need to promote and protect the welfare of citizens. By routinely deploying the language of personal responsibility over collective obligation, the UK government has acted in such a discretionary manner throughout the pandemic, showing itself capable of neglecting the shared interests of citizens through apathy, incompetence, or commitment to neoliberal ideology. Dependence on the arbitrary power of government in this way is incompatible with the enjoyment of republican liberty, and republican citizenship (Pettit, 1997, 36, 112).

In order to defuse the potential for such domination by the state, republicans argue that citizens should be able to continuously challenge and scrutinise the decisions and actions of those in power. This vigilant, contestatory model of democratic citizenship is designed to ensure that public decisions consider and track the interests of those impacted by them (Pettit, 1997, 184–184). Above and beyond existing modes of electoral democracy, citizens should have the formal capacity to challenge legislative, administrative, and judicial decisions through access to, and participation in, institutions such as parliamentary committees, formal bureaucratic inquiries, or quasi-judicial tribunals (ibid., 196).

Formal, institutionalised processes of contestation are not intended to grant individual citizens a veto over any and all public decisions they may personally dislike. Instead, they are intended to ensure that (i) public decisions are made in a procedurally fair and non-arbitrary way; and (ii) that these decisions are motivated by, and justified upon, a shared interest in the common good rather than any arbitrary whim, personal animus or casual disregard towards certain citizens (Pettit, 1997, 198). In other words, by actively engaging in democratic scrutiny of the state, its actions, and decisions, citizens can be confident that any interference inflicted by the state in their lives is non-arbitrary and therefore consistent with their individual freedom.

This model of active, vigilant citizenship contrasts markedly with the devaluation of democracy promoted by neoliberals. Rather than seeking to depoliticise areas of policy, abdicating responsibility to technocratic experts and elevating decisions beyond the purview of democratic scrutiny, the republican approach emphasises that meaningful contestation is essential to the enjoyment of freedom in a democracy.

On this view, democratic forums such as the citizens' panel convened by the Scottish Parliament during the pandemic can be seen as critically important to ensuring that the interventions and interference imposed by the state during the pandemic are made in a way that is non-arbitrary and non-dominating. Conversely, attempts by the UK government to depoliticise decision-making and evade meaningful democratic scrutiny undermine the legitimacy of these decisions, and inflict the very injuries to liberty that neoliberals claim to detest.

Certainly, in the context of a fast-moving and dynamic challenge such as a pandemic, action needs to be taken quickly and decisively. But such decisions also need to be made in a way that treats citizens as equal members of a democratic community, and in a way that promotes the common good rather than arbitrary personal interests. Fighting a pandemic is a collective effort, and one that can only be pursued effectively by rejecting the denuded, individualised model of citizenship offered by neoliberalism. Instead, the republican tradition of political thought urges us to fully embrace the opportunity for collective, and solidaristic, self-government through active engagement in the decision-making processes of the democratic state. Indeed, this alternative framework for governing the UK's pandemic response is necessary to truly protect the value of individual liberty in these extraordinary circumstances.

CONCLUSION

Because democracy presents as a threat to neoliberalism, neoliberalism has proven to be a threat to democracy. The neoliberal subject—the competent market actor—has been preferred to the democratic subject—the politically active citizen. The consequence has been devastating. Representative democracy and popular sovereignty have drifted apart, dangerously so. According to British political scientists Roger Eatwell and Matthew Goodwin (2018), democracy today is suffering on account of 4d's; distrust of politicians, destruction of national identities, deprivation and a sense of being left behind, and dis-alignment of political parties from their bases. The social compact between states and citizens required to mount an effective public health response to COVID-19 is simply no longer there. The first job facing a neorepublican state will be to save democracy from elections (at least in their current form) and reconnect governments with the citizens they are supposed to serve. Such a state must counter the mutation of an already flawed liberal democracy into something worse—an illiberal democracy. To build a more resilient UK, we need polities that are owned by all of the people for all of the people and not simply by a majority for a majority, or worse still a minority for a minority.

REFERENCES

Audickas, L. et al. (2019). *Membership of UK political parties.* https://commonslibrary.parliament.uk/research-briefings/sn05125/. Accessed 18 August 2021.

BBC News. (2021). Covid inquiry: When will it happen and how does it work? https://www.bbc.co.uk/news/explainers-57085964. Accessed 28 Dec 2021.

Brown, W. (2005). *Edgework: Critical essays on knowledge and politics.* Princeton University Press.

Brown, W. (2015). *Undoing the demos: Neoliberalism's stealth revolution*. Zone Books.

Burnham, P. (2001). New Labour and the politics of depoliticization. *British Journal of Politics and International Relations, 3*(2), 127–149.

Department for Business, Energy & Industrial Strategy. (2020). *Trade union membership, UK 1995–2019: Statistical bulletin*. https://assets.publishing. service.gov.uk/government/uploads/system/uploads/attachment_data/file/887740/Trade-union-membership-2019-statistical-bulletin.pdf. Accessed 18 Aug 2021.

Eatwell, R., & Goodwin, M. (2018). *National populism: The revolt against liberal democracy*. Pelican.

Evans, J. (2021). From stay at home, stay alert and back to stay at home: How government's lockdown messaging changed over the last year. https://www. itv.com/news/2021-03-21/from-stay-at-home-stay-alert-and-back-to-stay-at-home-how-governments-lockdown-messaging-changed-over-the-last-year. Accessed 28 Dec 2021.

Exeter, D., Paynter, J., & Bullen, C. (2020). Going hard and going early in New Zealand: The "team of 5 million" unites against COVID-19. https://www. liverpool.ac.uk/media/livacuk/publicpolicyamppractice/covid-19/PB024. pdf. Accessed 28 Dec 2021.

Gallo, E. (2021). Three varieties of authoritarian neoliberalism: Rule by the experts, the people, the leader. *Competition & Change*, 1–21.

Hacker, J. (2006). *The great risk shift: The new economic insecurity and the decline of the American dream*. Oxford University Press.

Hall, P. A., & Soskice, D. (Eds.). (2001). *Varieties of capitalism: The institutional foundations of comparative advantage*. OUP.

Harvey, D. (2005). *A brief history of neoliberalism*. Oxford University Press.

James, T. (2018). Chapter 2.4: Are UK elections conducted with integrity, with sufficient turnout? In P. Dunleavy, et al. (Eds.), *The UK's changing democracy* (pp.78–89). LSE Press.

Johnson, B. (2020, December 16). Prime Minister's statement on coronavirus (COVID-19). https://www.gov.uk/government/speeches/prime-ministers-statement-on-coronavirus-covid-19-16-december-2020c. Accessed 28 Dec 2021.

Joseph Rowntree Foundation. (2020). *UK poverty 2019/20*. Joseph Rowntree Foundation.

Kettell, S., & Kerr, P. (2021). 'Guided by the science': (De)politicising the UK government's response to the coronavirus crisis. *The British Journal of Politics and International Relations, 24*(1), 11–30.

Mudge, S. L. (2008). What is neo-liberalism? *Socio-Economic Review, 6*, 703–731.

Munck, R. (2005). Neoliberalism and politics, and the politics of neoliberalism. In A. Saad-Filho, & D. Johnston (Eds.), *Neoliberalism: A critical reader* (pp. 60–69). Pluto Press.

National Audit Office [NAO]. (2016). *Benefit sanctions*. National Audit Office

Näsström, S., & Kalm, S. (2015). A democratic critique of precarity. *Global Discourse, 5*(4), 556–573.

Nice, A. (2020). Extraordinary coronavirus restrictions on personal freedom require proper parliamentary scrutiny. https://www.instituteforgovernment. org.uk/blog/coronavirus-restrictions-parliamentary-scrutiny. Accessed 28 Dec 2021.

Pettit, P. (1996). Freedom as anti-power. *Ethics, 106*(3), 576–604.

Pettit, P. (1997). *Republicanism: A theory of freedom and government*. Oxford University Press.

Standing, G. (2011). *The precariat: The new dangerous class*. Bloomsbury.

The Scottish Parliament. (2021). Citizens' panel convened to discuss Scotland Covid-19 restrictions and strategy. https://archive2021.parliament.scot/new sandmediacentre/116952.aspx. Accessed 28 Dec 2021.

Thorsen, D. E. (2010). The neoliberal challenge: What is neoliberalism? *Contemporary Readings in Law and Social Justice, 2*(2), 188–214.

Tomasi, J. (2012). *Free market fairness*. Princeton University Press.

Trades Union Congress [TUC]. (2021). Sick pay that works. https://www.tuc. org.uk/research-analysis/reports/sick-pay-works. Accessed 28 Dec 2021.

Vallier, K. (2021). Neoliberalism. https://plato.stanford.edu/archives/sum 2021/entries/neoliberalism/. Accessed 28 Dec 2021.

Wright, S., Fletcher, D. R., & Stewart, A. B. R. (2020). Punitive benefit sanctions, welfare conditionality, and the social abuse of unemployed people in Britain: Transforming claimants into offenders? *Social Policy & Administration, 54*(2), 278–294.

CHAPTER 7

An Unequal Pandemic: Neoliberalism, Variegated Vulnerability, and Uneven Disease Burdens

Abstract Free market capitalism both actively produces social and spatial inequalities and opposes state intervention to remediate these inequalities. For neoliberals, inequalities and injustices should not be conflated and in any case, it is neither desirable nor necessary for the state to proactively intervene to rebalance differences and divergence. Whilst the United Kingdom (UK) displays below-average levels of wealth and income inequalities globally, it presents as one of the most unequal and polarised of the OECD countries and in particular has the most unequal space economy in the OECD world, suffering from stark regional inequalities and an acute North–South divide. Perhaps most importantly, under and because of neoliberalism, social and spatial inequalities have significantly increased across the past 40 years. This development has mediated the UK's encounter with COVID-19—directly and indirectly. Wealth and income inequalities—including and in particular growing inequalities and relative deprivation—are central progenitors of health inequalities, public distrust of government and the erosion of social capital and community cohesion—all of which have increased vulnerability, at least for some social strata. In a vicious cycle, COVID-19 in turn has aggravated, social and spatial inequalities in wealth, income, and health in the UK.

Keywords Inequalities · Trust · Relative inequalities · Health inequalities · Co-morbidities · Social capital · Social justice · Spatial justice

© The Author(s), under exclusive license to Springer Nature Switzerland AG 2022
M. Boyle et al., *COVID-19 and the Case Against Neoliberalism*,
https://doi.org/10.1007/978-3-031-18935-7_7

Introduction

Free market capitalism both actively produces social and spatial inequalities and opposes state intervention to remediate these inequalities For neoliberals, inequalities are not in themselves injustices and in any event, it is neither desirable nor necessary for the state to proactively intervene to rebalance difference and divergence. Whilst the UK displays below average levels of wealth and income inequalities globally, it presents as one of most unequal and polarised of the OECD countries and in particular has the most unequal space economy in the OECD world, suffering from stark regional inequalities and an acute North–South divide. Perhaps most importantly, under and because of neoliberalism, social and spatial inequalities have significantly increased across the past 40 years. This development has mediated the UK's encounter with COVID-19—directly and indirectly. Wealth and income inequalities—including and in particular *growing* inequalities and relative deprivation—are central progenitors of health inequalities, public distrust of government, and the erosion of social capital and community cohesion—all of which have increased vulnerability, at least for some social strata. In a vicious cycle, COVID-19 in turn has aggravated, social and spatial inequalities in wealth, income, and health in the UK.

Neoliberalism and (Growing) Wealth and Income Inequalities

A perversity lies at the core of neoliberalism; whilst market fundamentalism actively produces, and indeed as Neil Smith (1984) has demonstrated necessarily depends upon, the existence of, social and spatial inequalities in wealth and income, neoliberal philosophy promotes the view that it is both morally wrong and technically unnecessary for governments to seek to intervene to remediate these inequalities. The result is a damaging and incredulous cycle of market liberalisation followed by growing inequalities followed by the preferred panacea—more aggressive neoliberalism redux!

Neoliberalism resists the premise of redistributive egalitarianism, denies the concept of social justice and rejects ideas of solidarity looking to destroy social institutions, such as trade unions, and the public provision of housing, utilities, or healthcare (Hanlon, 2015). This aversion to the political remediation of the socioeconomic inequalities thrown up and/or generated by capitalist society can be seen to stem from the particular view of individual liberty to which neoliberals subscribe. Recall that neoliberals hold that protecting each individual's natural right to personal sovereignty and self-ownership—the capacity to act, chose, contract, and exchange with others as each sees fit—should be paramount. This means that the state, or any other agent for that matter, may not interfere with the actions or decisions of individuals without compromising individual liberty, even if that interference is required to improve the lives of others, advance collective welfare, or deliver greater material equality.

The neoliberal view of justice instead looks backwards, to the history of how unequal distributions have arisen, rather than evaluating the probity or permissibility of any distribution as it exists in the present. So long as inequality is the result of free and fair exchange, where nobody has been coerced into parting with their private resources or making decisions nonvoluntarily, then it is considered to be no business of the state to interfere with this outcome. More than this, any attempt to artificially create and maintain a particular pattern or distribution of equality is seen to necessarily undermine individual liberty in ways that are philosophically unacceptable to neoliberals. Instead, the neoliberal state's primary duty is not to extend and maintain greater equality between citizens, it is to extend and maintain the bases of free and fair exchange, namely, open markets. The state ought not to impose some perfectionist idea of the good on others, and nor should the state seek to maintain this idea of the good at the expense of individuals' self-ownership. Interfering with "capitalist acts between consenting adults" (Nozick, 1974, 163), would violate the individual freedom to choose how best to live one's own life. So long as freedom as non-interference is maintained, neoliberals are likely to be entirely relaxed about rising inequalities. Indeed, these are an acceptable price to pay for liberty.

The libertarian political philosopher Robert Nozick articulates this position in what he calls 'the entitlement theory of justice' (1974, 151). What matters, according to this theory, is how a given distribution of resources has come about, not whether it meets the standards of some externally imposed (egalitarian) ideal of distributive justice. Nozick summarises this idea, stating that "Whatever arises from a just situation by just steps is itself just" (ibid.). By contrast, any attempt to create and maintain some ideal distribution or pattern would require us to continually override the freedom of individuals to use their private resources how they see fit, they would be prevented from acting for themselves to a certain extent. Crucially, Nozick suggests that it is a fact of freedom that "Not everyone wants the same things, or wants them as strongly" (1974, 249). To treat people as unable to make these decisions for themselves would undermine their natural right to self-ownership and self-direction. The state ought not to impose some perfectionist idea of the good on others, and nor should the state seek to maintain this idea of the good at the expense of individuals' self-ownership. Interfering with "capitalist acts between consenting adults" (Nozick, 1974, 163), would violate the individual freedom to choose how best to live one's own life.

This logic can also be extended to health and wellbeing. Some people may choose to value their personal health, and they should be free to pursue this value through their personal choices and actions in an open market. For example, they may choose to prioritise purchasing healthy food options, even if these are more expensive, or they may choose to pay for regular visits to a private doctor. Nevertheless, on this view, it would be unjust to impose this perfectionist idea of the good on the whole of society as this would constrain the freedom of others who may wish to pursue ideas and interests that matter more to them than their personal health and wellbeing, for example enjoying tobacco, alcohol, fatty foods, etc. So long as health inequalities are the outcome of non-coerced, voluntaristic choices by sovereign economic agents, then the outcomes—no matter how unequal—must be considered the just outcome of their freely-made actions and decisions over time. In contrast, launching public health interventions on behalf of the state—for example, against consumption of tobacco, alcohol, or fatty foods—would be seen as imposing illegitimate, and patronising, constraints on individuals' freedom to choose and act how they wish, compromising individual liberty.

By dint of problems of its own making, this defence of the market as a moral institution is increasingly becoming difficult to accept.

French Economist Thomas Piketty has played a central role in the development of the World Inequalities Database (WID), the establishment of the World Inequalities Lab and the publication of the World Inequality Report (2020, and more recently updated and expanded in 2022). He has also played a central role in mining the WID and rendering intelligible the trends that this database is now revealing. Piketty's ground-breaking book titled *Capital in the Twenty-First Century*, 2019 sequel titled *Capital and Ideology* and 2022 capstone book titled *A Brief*

History of Inequality have come to stand as consequential interventions in the global debate on neoliberalism and inequality.

Piketty charts the historical evolution of inequalities in wealth (capital and financial assets [savings, property, bonds, gold, stocks, pensions, inheritances]) and income inequalities (wages, bonuses, salaries, dividends, interest on savings, state benefits, pensions, rent, etc.), demonstrating that both have been widening since the early 1980s. On the basis of the ideas of r (the rate of return on capital) and g (the rate of economic growth) and the formula $r > g$, Piketty argues that capitalism is anatomically wired to ensure that wealth grows faster than the economy. Income returns to the owners of capital (wealth) at a higher rate than it does to the rest of society and in consequence inequalities grow over time. Historical exceptions to this formula are aberrations.

Piketty sketches the following periodisation:

- *The rise of 'vulgar capitalism' (1800-World War I and the roaring 1920s)*. During this period, patrimonial capitalism reigned and a comparatively limited number of wealthy people owned an increasingly larger portion of the wealth of nations and through inheritance, passed on this privilege to their heirs. $r > g$ and income accrued to the wealthy disproportionately, making them incrementally wealthier over time. Within country, inequalities widened dramatically.

- *Rewarding work not wealth (World War I, the 1930s Great Depression, World War II, and 1945–1975)*. Only a burst of rapid growth (from technological progress or rising population) or government intervention can lead to $g > r$. World War I, World War II, and the welfare Keynesianism era 1945–1975 combined to serve as one such period. Damage inflicted by war reduced the share of total wealth held by elites. Meanwhile, state redistributive policies and rising wages meant that the rate of return accruing to labour exceeded the rate of return to capital. A convergence in income inequalities and, in consequence, wealth inequalities was the result.

- *Wealth is back! The rise of neoliberalism (from the early 1980s)*. With the ascent of the dominant neoliberal economic model, the elite has mounted a full-fronted action to recover their lost advantage; wealth and not work has become again a key progenitor of income, $r > g$, and catching up has ceded to falling behind. Wealth is back! Whilst inequalities in income and wealth have not yet returned to that which prevailed during the age of 'vulgar capitalism', they are growing again. A potent and destabilising new geography of discontent has emerged, especially in left behind rustbelt cities, giving rise to nationalistic political populisms.

Piketty's work is hugely valuable but perhaps under-specified. Surely the veracity of the formula $r > g$ is a product of historical and political forces and is not an immutable fact inherent in capitalism? Is not wealth inequality a proximate determinant of trends in income inequalities rather than a fundamental progenitor of these inequalities? What political struggles and victories lie beneath patterns of r and g historically? In fact inequalities in health arise as a result of socio-political factors—market fundamentalism—that lead to unequal distributions of power, money, and resources between different population groups and social classes.

Reframed thus, Piketty's narrative arc captures almost exactly the history of wealth and income inequalities in the UK. Still benefiting from the legacy effects of Keynesian redistributive policies, as measured by the WID Palma Index of Inequality (confirmed by the UNHDRO Palma Index of Inequality and the World Bank GINI Index of Inequality), the UK displays below average levels of inequality globally. But it is burdened by above-average levels of inequality within the OECD group. Moreover, wealth and income inequalities have significantly increased in the past 40 years (Figs. 7.1, 7.2 and 7.3).

At the close of the Victorian era, and at a time when imperial and urban industrial Britain lay at the centre of the world capitalist economy, the UK was one the most unequal countries on earth. World War I, the 1930s depression and World War II, were followed by decolonisation and the rise, post-war, of a high growth Fordist economy and Keynesian welfare state. The top 1% and top 10% of the population by wealth secured a smaller share of the national product whilst the bottom 50% of the population became comparatively enriched. Wealth inequalities began to narrow. The rise of Thatcherism and supply side monetary economics in the early 1980s, however, reversed these gains and once again the wealthy began to accrue more than an equal share of the national product. Successive British governments have restructured the economy by shifting away from heavy industries and manufacturing towards finance and services leading to unemployment and poverty in affected communities. It has also favoured privatisation and deregulation redistributing wealth in the favour of the rich not only leading to a lack of state capacity but also immensely widening inequalities. It has dismantled public welfare provision when

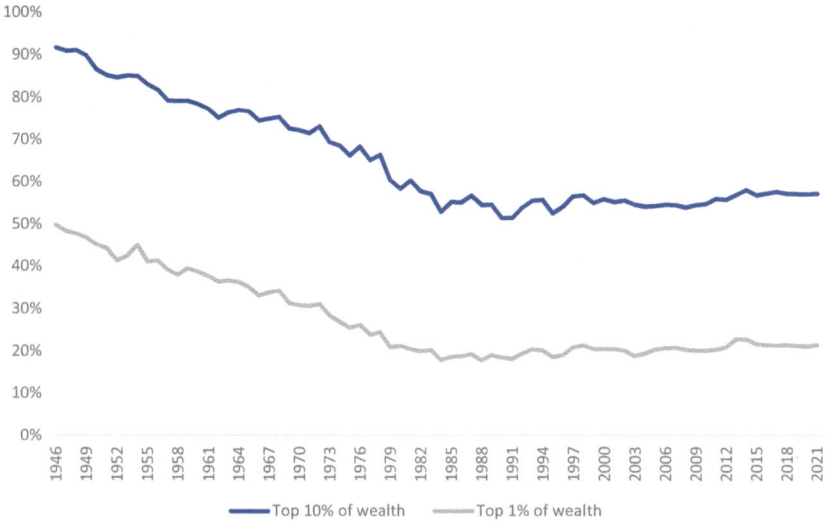

Fig. 7.1 % of total wealth held by the top 10% and top 1% in the UK 1945–2021 (*Source* World Inequalities Database https://wid.world/)

unemployment was at a high level increasing poverty (Hanlon, 2015). The neoliberal state of the UK has been efficiently advancing and maintaining the financial system of the country in the name of the free market whilst disregarding the poorest and most vulnerable people of society as beyond its responsibility.

In the UK and more specifically post-imperial England, this historical dynamic has etched an indelible imprint on the geography of the space economy, leaving a much-discussed North–South divide, although in reality spatial injustice and disparities in living standards are distributed in complex ways at a variety of scales throughout the entire country. The mid-twentieth century demise of the UK's metropolitan dominance over what has been referred to as an 'imperial world economy' or 'old international division of labour' paved the way for an age of globalisation and a 'new international division of labour' marked by: (i) a consolidation of transnational corporation headquarters, financial institutions and producer services in London and the South-East, and in consequence an accelerated growth of the UK's capital city as a cosmopolitan

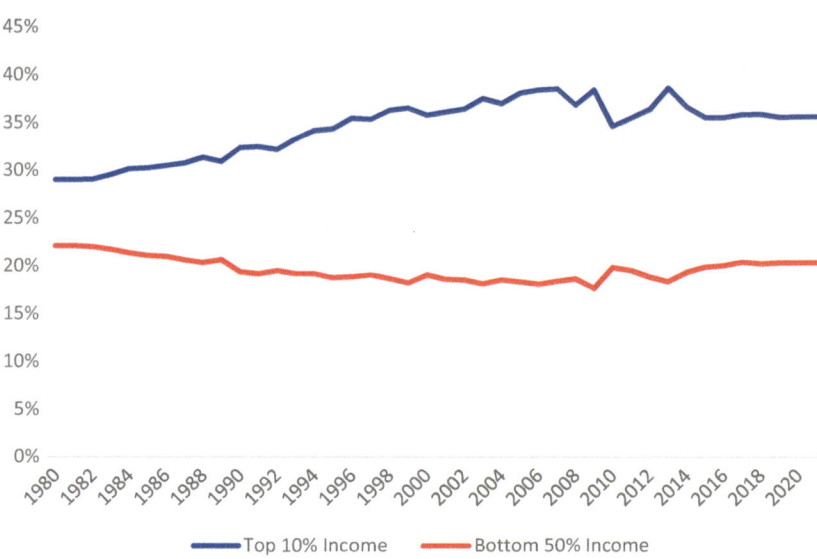

Fig. 7.2 % of national income accruing to the top 10% and bottom 50% in the UK 1980–2021 (*Source* World Inequalities Database https://wid.world/)

'alpha' global city, and (ii) an increasing globalisation of many industrial processes, with the concomitant deindustrialisation of the UK's once vibrant imperial industrial workshops and port cities, in particular the city-regions of northern England, and capital flight as a result a comparative lack of prosperity and opportunity. Within London itself, world city status has come with unprecedented levels of local socio-spatial polarisation. The global financial crisis and attendant period of neoliberalism redux and austerity (2008–2015) have sealed the deal; growing the size of the British population living in poverty and cutting adrift more starkly those with low incomes and those living in deprived communities. Uneven geographic development has been accelerated by a highly centralised state architecture and a disposition to favour a spatially blind national investment strategy which wittingly and unwittingly has reinforced and aggravated socio-spatial polarisation. And the considered judgement is that Brexit will only serve to aggravate socio-spatial inequalities across the UK (McCann, 2016, 2020; McCann et al., 2022).

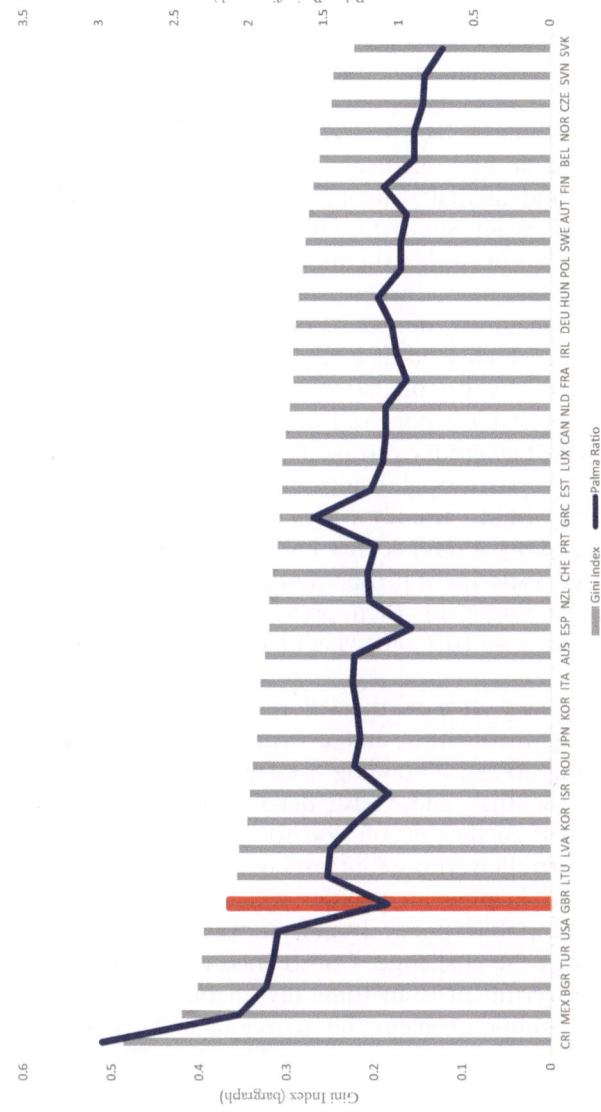

Fig. 7.3 Inequality: The UK in the context of the OECD world (*Source* OECD https://data.oecd.org/)

Would evangelists of neoliberalism accept the charge that liberalised markets may well lift people and places out of poverty but they both actively produce, and lack the ability to remediate, social and spatial inequalities in wealth and income? Perhaps, some would! Neoliberalism is a growth machine after all. Is it not better to be absolutely rich and relatively unequal than absolutely poor but relatively equal?

Overlooking for now the fact that across the past forty years neoliberalism has achieved at best mediocre rates of growth, infact such a riposte would be fundamentally incommensurable with neoliberalism's root promise. From Adam Smith to Friedrich Von Hayek and Milton Friedman, the claim has been that the hidden hand of the market confers not only optimum economic efficiency but also 'moral sentiment': the market itself and alone and by dint of its operational logic, would fix any negative externalities which it itself birthed. Liberalized markets would both: (a) increase the wealth of nations and transform the quality of human life, lifting the world's poor out of poverty and; (b) correct over time diverging levels of economic prosperity and geographical inequalities in wealth and income across social divides and geographical scales. Unsustainable inequalities would naturally wither over time to be replaced by shared prosperity and social and spatial justice. That market fundamentalism has sponsored a species of prosperity that is wired to render shared prosperity structurally impossible then, presents as an existential threat to neoliberalism's worldview. To (somewhat) pass (a) but fail (b) is to fail overall.

In spite of becoming alive to the failures of neoliberalism and the dangers of widening inequalities and a divided society, despite much chatter over 'levelling up', and 'building back better' and in spite of much braggadocio about Scottish and Welsh devolution, a settled Northern Ireland Assembly, and further devolution to English combined authorities and a 'Northern Powerhouse', there is little cause to hope that widening wealth and income inequalities will be remediated any time soon. Currently, the public policy agenda looks hopelessly inadequate given the enormity of the challenge. Constrained by neoliberal ideology, arguably the UK government is anatomically unable to take the kind of decisive measures a public problem this tenacious and wicked demands (UK2070, 2020).

Wealth and Income Inequalities in the UK and Uneven Social and Spatial COVID-19 Burdens

Why might inequalities matter in the production of variegated vulnerability and exposure to harm from COVID-19, for people and places?

Globally, relationships between wealth and income inequalities, uneven geographic development, and socially and spatially variegated encounters with COVID-19 are clearly complex. Between-country variations in COVID-19 outcomes can only be partially explained by the scale of within country inequalities. Russia, countries with the highest levels of within-country inequality in the OECD (United States, Chile, Colombia), and in the Global South (across the whole of Latin America (especially Brazil), India, and South Africa, have indeed often endured the worst of the pandemic. But in East Asia (especially China and South Korea) and Australia, growing inequalities have not jeopardised or even-tempered efforts to suppress COVID-19. Meanwhile, a significant number of African countries have avoided the worst of COVID-19 notwithstanding their very high levels of inequality. Notwithstanding their comparatively lower levels of inequality, Belgium, Slovenia, and the Czech Republic have all borne a disproportionate disease burden.

Might we conclude that within-country inequalities should be ruled out as a causal variable in the production of vulnerability? Absolutely not! What matters is the specific workings of market fundamentalism in particular countries; we need to understand in granular detail local processes and trends and the meaning and implications of widening wealth and income inequalities locally. In the UK, absolute inequalities matter—many communities in post-austerity Britain face an absolute scarcity of essential resources; food, fuel, and adequate housing. But as Wilkinson and Pickett (2010, 2020, 15) have shown time and again, it is relative deprivation and the internalisation of psychosocial wounding that does the damage: "The big idea is that what matters in determining mortality and health in a society is less the overall wealth of that society and more how evenly wealth is distributed. The more equally wealth is distributed the better the health of that society". Coming after thirty years of economic growth and enhanced sharing of prosperity, forty years of neoliberalism, weak economic growth and widening social and spatial inequalities have fractured British society to the core.

Figures 7.4 and 7.5 profile confirmed COVID-19 death rates and excess death rates in the UK by deprivation decile. It is uncontroversial to state that in the case of the UK, COVID-19 has preyed on growing inequalities disproportionately impacting poor communities living in the country's most deprived deciles—Black, Asian, and Minority Ethnic (BAME) communities, rustbelt deindustrialised places and those living in exceptional precarity including homeless people, prisoners, and sex workers (Bambra et al., 2020; Suleman et al., 2021). Not only are COVID-19 death rates higher in more deprived communities but these communities also have borne more excess deaths, that is excess deaths in excess of the number of excess deaths due to COVID-19. The implication is that these communities have not only been less able to stop COVID-19, these have also been unable to stop COVID-19 from bequeathing spillover negative health outcomes.

In the specific context of the UK, why might inequalities matter in the production of variegated vulnerability and exposure to harm from COVID-19, for people and places?

In the case of the UK, a number of direct causal connections between inequalities and COVID-19 outcomes are immediately obvious. Wealth and income inequalities mean that environmental and individual resources are distributed variably, resulting in differences in the quality and availability of employment, housing, transport, access to services, and social and cultural resources. It has been easier for certain societal groups to protect their health whilst other population groups were disproportionately negatively impacted. People in lower income households and those living in areas of deprivation were more exposed to the virus in part because they were unable to work from home, were engaged in more hazardous front-line public facing service occupations, live in overcrowded housing, lack easy access to green space, suffer disproportionately from digital poverty, and were most reliant upon public transport. Additionally, to a meaningful degree, vulnerable groups had to self-isolate due to the pandemic and experienced escalating poverty and loss of employment, reporting therein much higher levels of anxiety subsequent to the outbreak of the pandemic (Wang et al., 2020). Women were hardest hit by working-from-home measures and school closures, with many juggling paid work, home-schooling, and housework, whilst single mothers faced additional issues such as disproportionate poverty, withdrawal of support services, and social isolation (Beveridge, 2020): The extent of COVID-19 deaths in long-term care homes (LTCH)

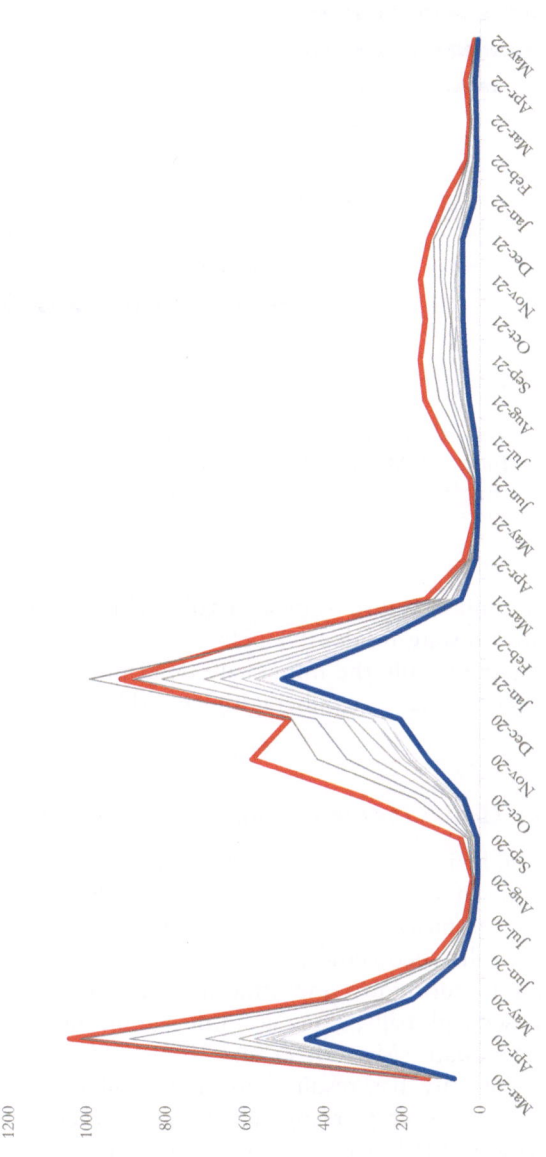

Fig. 7.4 Age standardised COVID 19 death rates by deprivation decile 2020–2022. Decile 1 (most deprived) Red, Decile 10 (least deprived) Blue (*Source* UK ONS https://www.ons.gov.uk/)

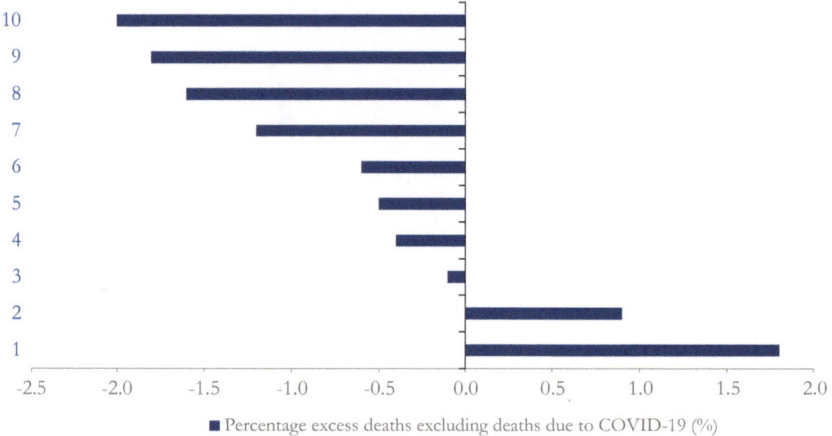

Fig. 7.5 Percentage excess deaths that is deaths in excess of those caused by COVID-19 directly by Index of Multiple Deprivation decile, registered March 2020–December 2021, England. Decile 1 (most deprived), Decile 10 (least deprived) (*Source* UK ONS https://www.ons.gov.uk/)

points to a widespread moral failure to protect vulnerable elderly groups, especially those reliant on state-funded LTCHs.

But this is to focus upon only the immediate determinants of uneven disease burdens. A deeper layer of neoliberal logics and legacies must also be considered.

Underlying Health Inequalities and Co-Morbidities

Because COVID-19 linked co-morbidities vary between populations, so too there exists an uneven social geography of vulnerability to COVID-19. One of the most pernicious manifestations of wealth and income inequalities is that of health inequalities.

Whilst inequalities in morbidity and mortality in the UK may be at lower levels than seen globally, rates are still significant and as the 2020 Marmot report update (Marmot et al., 2020—see also Marmot, 2010), a decade of austerity has resulted in an overall decline in life expectancy in the UK and ever growing health inequalities (Fig. 7.6). Public Health England's 2014 inquiry into health inequalities in the North of England—*Due North: Report of the Inquiry on Health Equity for the North*—observed that the gap between the North and the South of England has been widening for over four decades and under five different governments leading to 1.5 million excess premature deaths in the North (Whitehead et al., 2014). In Scotland, the Glasgow Centre for Population Health (GCPH) has attributed much sharper health inequalities that can be accounted for by deprivation to both a 'Glasgow effect' (context (place/neighborhood) and not just composition (socioeconomic profile) matters) and a 'political affect' (the differential impact of austerity on post-industrial cites) (Schoefield et al., 2020). As the Cambridge multi-morbidity project has shown people living in chronic poverty and precarity and dwelling in disadvantaged neighbourhoods have higher rates of almost all of the known underlying clinical risk factors that increase the severity and mortality of COVID-19, including hypertension, diabetes, asthma, chronic obstructive pulmonary disease (COPD), heart disease, liver disease, renal disease, cancer, cardiovascular disease, obesity, and smoking. Bambra et al. (2020) conclude that COVID-19 then, forms part of a synergistic epidemic or syndemic (Singer, 2009)—adding a further layer of health inequalities on top of and interacting with—prior layers.

Public (Mis)trust of Government and Inability to Command a Social Licence for Public Health Interventions

Many liberal democratic OECD countries have recorded higher cases and deaths per capita than more authoritarian countries such as China, Vietnam, Egypt, Saudi Arabia, Nigeria, Malawi, and the Democratic Republic of Congo. This has perhaps been unsurprising given that enforced lockdowns, contact tracing technology, mandatory mask-wearing, etc., require a degree of coercion and preparedness to forgo certain personal liberties. To be as effective, democratic polities need to command a very high level of public confidence. Surveys measuring public trust in government suggest that democratic governments are failing miserably to inspire trust and loyalty from citizens. The UK government consistently ranks amongst the least trusted (in surveys such as those undertaken by the OECD, the Edelman Trust, and the World Values Survey WVS), with polls averaging at around 40% trust. A schism has opened between representative democratic institutions and popular sovereignty which has in turn almost certainly mitigated against the capacity of democratic polities to implement stringent containment measures. Curiously, whilst not alone, populist governments seem to

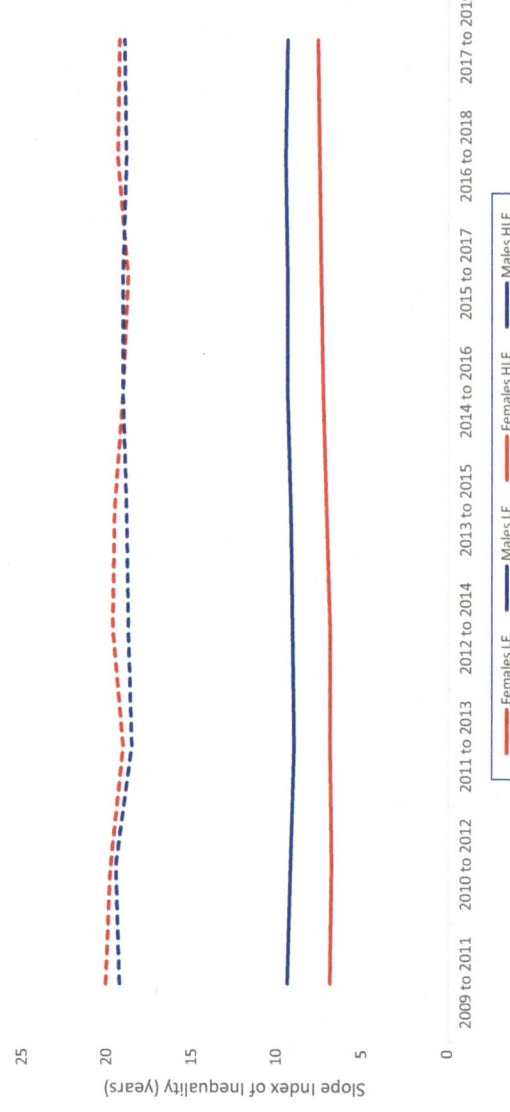

Fig. 7.6 Slope Index of Inequality in life expectancy and healthy life expectancy at birth 2009–2019 by gender

have presided over particularly poor outcomes: Trump in the United States, Johnson in the UK, Bolsonaro in Brazil, Modi in India, Orban in Hungary, and Erdoğan in Turkey. These movements tend to come freighted with (ill-founded, for the most part) assertions about the need to reclaim citizens' liberties and rights from the state, and the proclivity to privilege individual freedoms over state mandates might be part of the explanation. Asian democracies such as South Korea, Taiwan and Japan are exceptions to the rule; where particular local attitudes towards authority, community and compliance may explain the better performance of these democratic polities. Meanwhile, countries like Australia and New Zealand have demonstrated a capacity to gain a democratic license to limit personal liberties, at least for a period.

The Uneven Impact of COVID-19 is Cooted in the Demise of Social Cohesion

Countries where social capital, solidarity, mutuality, and reciprocity have been eroded and depleted most will suffer disproportionate harm. Historically, the work which place-based communities have done in protecting vulnerable people in times of need and strengthening resilience for all has been critical. Alas, forty years of neoliberalism and a decade of austerity appears to have dismantled the complex webs of connective lines and tissues braided within and between communities at myriad scales. Much has been made of the decline of community in western societies; in particular, the erosion of trust between people and depletion of social capital (a finding repeatedly confirmed by the World Values Surveys series, WVS). Responsibility for the provision of social care has shifted from families and communities to governments. When enacted without a sense of solidarity, such 'caring from a distance' can be overly transactional and can present as impoverished, disembodied, cool, and detached. Countries that have both preserved strong communities and endured COVID-19 better include the Nordic countries, Australia, China, Vietnam, and New Zealand. In contrast, countries that have witnessed both a decline in social trust and been especially vulnerable to COVID-19 include the United States, the United Kingdom, France, Spain, and the majority of Latin American states. But while most African countries are considered relatively bereft of social capital, they appear to have weathered the pandemic better than a number of countries that report relatively healthy stocks of social capital such as India, Russia, South Africa, Saudi Arabia, and to a degree Canada and Germany. But once again it is changing levels—and changing relative inequalities, rather than absolute levels of social trust and community solidarity that does most damage.

Nondomination as an Egalitarian Ideal

According to Piketty (2020), there is nothing inevitable or innocent about inequality; it is not an innate species condition but instead a structural feature of capitalism, further moderated by political choices. Piketty coins the phrase 'inequality regime' to understand the justification [used] for the structure of inequality and also the institutions—the legal system, the educational system, the fiscal system—that help sustain a certain level of inequity in a given society. He accepts the need for and the advantages of private wealth and the value of a certain degree of inequality. But he argues that inequality has reached levels that are intolerable; they not only burden people living in both absolute and relative poverty, but they are bad for economic growth and sow the seeds of political disquiet. Growing inequalities have been centrally implicated in the rise of political populisms and nationalist political movements around the world and the emergence of a politics of anger and resentment amongst those who feel that they have been 'left behind' and languish in a dying 'rustbelt' condemned to 'managed decline'. Piketty's solution is a new participatory socialism predicated on economic democracy and the right of everyone to participate in the design, governance and regulation of the market economy. He proposes a series of 'confiscatory taxes' to be allocated to a new generation of Universal Basic Services, the establishment of a Universal Basic Income and the payment of a minimal Universal Inheritance.

Whilst generally sympathetic to Piketty's proposal, we chose here to approach the challenge of reducing wealth and income inequalities using the analytical tools of neorepublicanism. These tools do not align in any simple way with Piketty's 'participatory socialism' but we consider them to be cognate and capable of generating a productive conversation. By adopting a neorepublican view of freedom as non-domination, rather than non-interference, widening inequalities can instead be seen to pose a significant threat to individual liberty that the state ought to rectify. Inequality between citizens is not something that must be tolerated in order to maximise freedom, and nor must we necessarily sacrifice liberty in order to promote greater equality. On the republican view, inequalities can be understood to represent both a cause and consequence of domination in society. If our aim is to maximise freedom as non-domination we are required to proactively minimise the inequalities of power and resources that could enable some agents to dominate others.

Republican freedom as non-domination requires a context of "intersubjective equality" (Pettit, 1997, 64), in which agents are able to perceive of themselves as relating to others as equal citizens. The existence of power hierarchies in which one agent dominates others upsets this equality, "the power-victim cannot enjoy the psychological status of an equal: they are in a position where fear and deference will be the normal order of the day" (ibid.). As one extreme example, consider the kinds of relationship portrayed in the film *The Godfather*, in which the power of Marlon Brando's Don Corleone, with his capacity to command violence and coercion at will and with impunity, is so implicitly understood that he is able to make offers to those less powerful than him that, in turn, they literally cannot refuse. They know they must instead sycophantically bend to his every whim, or else suffer the potential consequences. By drawing on their unequal share of resources and power, individuals such as Don Corleone can dominate others, with a capacity to interfere arbitrarily in the lives of others in a way that is difficult to resist or repel. This capacity to dominate others, in turn, undermines the possibility of all citizens enjoying a shared status of intersubjective equality, enabling certain individuals to stand above the rest.

The power imbalances enabled by social or economic inequality between citizens must therefore be seen as incompatible with republican liberty, which requires individuals to be secured against the potential for arbitrary or discretionary power to be exercised over them. Philip Pettit illustrates this point, arguing that freedom as non-domination ensures that individuals are able to meet what he calls the 'eyeball test': "They can look others in the eye without reason for the fear or deference that a power of interference might inspire; they can walk tall and assume the public status, objective and subjective, of being equal in this regard with the best...The satisfaction of the test would mean for each person that others were unable, in the received phrase, to interfere at will and with impunity in their affairs" (2012, 84). Where this eyeball test is not met, freedom cannot be found. Inequality enables some to wield power over others, and the presence of this domination in turn undermines the potential for all to enjoy the status of free and equal citizenship.

For republicans, we must utilise the full potential of the state to promote this equality of standing between citizens, ensuring that suitable legal and institutional mechanisms are in place to enable each individual to meet the eyeball test with others (Pettit, 2012, 87–89). Should the state fail to provide all citizens with equally robust protection against arbitrary power, then it would, itself, come to represent a source of domination in its own right; one that wields the power to discretionarily permit the domination of some and not others in society. For this reason, Pettit argues that freedom as non-domination must be understood as an inherently egalitarian good, one that needs to be distributed more or less equally by the state in order for it to be maximally realised (1997, 110–116; 2012, 90–91).

Recall that freedom as non-domination is a social and political status, one that is constituted by institutions that—"like the immunity produced by antibodies in the blood" (Pettit, 1997, 274)—determine one's capacity to reliably resist domination by others. In other words, republican liberty requires the presence of institutions that reduce and eliminate the power that certain agents would otherwise be able to wield over others arbitrarily (Pettit, 1996, 588–590). These institutions, like the neorepublican ideal of freedom as non-domination itself, are inherently egalitarian in nature. They would include a free and fair legal system that is applied equally and transparently to all in society, as well as institutions to regulate the power of those in economically or politically privileged positions from dominating others (ibid., 590–591). For example, Pettit suggests a suitably republican state would seek to equalise the relationship between employers and employees by promoting regulations that prevent employers from being able to terminate employment at will, and protect workers' rights to unionise and strike against poor conditions (2012, 115). Such institutions support the maintenance of intersubjective equality between citizens by ensuring that each is able to repel potential domination—not by luck or by skill—but by the presence of robust and reliable republican institutions.

Pettit, for one, suggests that republican liberty does not *necessarily* require the state to enforce material equality, that is equality of resources and opportunities, in the strictest sense (1997, 117–119). Nevertheless, he concedes that "the promotion of freedom as non-domination is likely in the actual world to require the reduction of material inequalities" (ibid., 118). This is because non-domination will require the institutional cultivation of socioeconomic independence (ibid., 158–163). This can be promoted through institutions that are "designed to enhance the day-to-day capacities...for example, measures ensuring universal education and universal access to culturally important services like transportation and communication" (Pettit, 1996, 591). Such empowering institutions would also include a right to welfare state measures such as sufficient social security, legal aid, and access to healthcare in order to prevent individuals ever becoming reliant on the good will or indifference of powerful agents—doctors, lawyers, welfare bureaucrats, etc.—in the event of misfortune (ibid., 592; 1997, 159–160). These kinds of institutional interventions are designed to promote, in Pettit's word, "equality in basic capabilities" (1996, 591), dampening the capacity of the privileged to utilise their resources to dominate the less privileged.

Elsewhere, Pettit has argued that the neorepublican political programme could additionally require a right to a basic income—a guaranteed minimum income paid universally and unconditionally by the state to all citizens on a periodic basis—that would function to equalise the distribution of power in society, and neutralise the capacity of wealthy agents to interfere at will and with impunity in the lives of the less wealthy. For example, Pettit writes:

> Suppose there are just a few employers and many available employees, and that times are hard. In those conditions I and those who like me will not be able to command a decent wage: a wage that will enable us to function properly in society. And in those conditions it will be equally true that we would be defenseless against our employers' petty abuse or their power to arbitrarily dismiss us. Other protections, such as those that strong trade unions might provide, are possible against such alien control. But the most effective of all protections, and one that should complement other measures available, would be one's ability to leave employment and fall back on a basic wage available unconditionally from the state (Pettit, 2007, 5).

In arguing for such protective, regulatory, and empowering institutions and mechanisms that act to insure and insulate individuals against the potential for domination by those with greater power and resources, neorepublicans show that the pursuit of liberty and greater equality need not be in tension as neoliberals would suggest. Minimising the capacity of certain agents to dominate others requires the state to defuse the power that material resources and opportunities could grant them over others. Simultaneously, cultivating a context of intersubjective equality between citizens requires proactive efforts to narrow socioeconomic inequalities, ensuring all citizens have access to sufficient goods and services such as healthcare.

Crucially, there is no reason, on republican grounds, to reject the kinds of coercive redistribution of wealth necessary to afford such egalitarian measures. As Pettit explains, "the taxation needed to support a social security system need not count as domination, and need not count therefore as a serious assault on people's liberty; it may represent a suitably controlled, and so nonarbitrary form of government interference" (2010, 51). Such interference is not only permissible, but necessary in order to equalise the power relations between citizens, insulating them against the potential for being dominated by others, and insuring them against the risk of falling reliant on the mercy of powerful actors.

In this respect neorepublicanism offers a broadly social democratic political programme (Pettit, 2010, 49), utilising the capacity of the state to promote greater equality between citizens not in spite of individual liberty, but in pursuit of it. So long as the state is constituted in a way that it does not represent a source of domination in its own right, it may legitimately seek to establish the kinds of public institutional mechanisms that function to defuse and neutralise inequalities in power and resources, in order to dampen their social and political consequences.

From the standpoint of neorepublican theory, then, we can view widening socioeconomic inequalities, such as those witnessed across the UK over recent decades, as absurd, unnecessary, and incompatible with the promotion of individual liberty. The neoliberal state has feigned impotence, suggesting that cuts to the welfare state and an abandonment of social security were unavoidable, and that the inequalities these have unleashed are somehow inevitable. As a particular conception of freedom as non-interference, has become normalised and valorised through neoliberal political philosophy and public policy practice, we have lost sight of the extent to which intersubjective equality between citizens is a necessary precondition for achieving a free society. And we have lost sight of the potential of the democratic state to maintain the social, economic, and political foundations of this equality: the social democratic institutions that formed the heart of the UK's post-war consensus.

The welfare state, with its commitment to a well-funded and effective social security system, National Health Service, public education, council housing, and so on functioned, in principle, to equalise the relations between citizens, insulating individuals from dominating power. They also had the corollary effect of equalising material outcomes, reducing the gaps in health, wealth, and quality of life that had typified pre-war Britain. Far from representing the patronising and stifling grip of the so-called nanny state, the proactive welfare state can be seen as the necessary institutional foundation for counter-domination, giving individuals the capacity to interact with the world from a secure position of freedom and equality with others.

For neorepublicans, the corrosion of the post-war UK's social democratic foundations can be understood as a needless act of self-harm, one that served neither the cause of liberty or equality. Citizens have not been made freer by a system in which they are poorer, less healthy, and less empowered than others. Inequality is neither the rational nor just outcome of free market preferences. It is the failure of a neoliberal state to maintain the conditions of intersubjective equality necessary for citizens to enjoy freedom together, where socioeconomic disparities don't automatically translate into a capacity to dominate others. This is clear, none more so, than in the realm of public health. As health inequalities have widened, following a grim social gradient that has left the poorest and most deprived citizens most at risk of poor health and early death, this should have been recognised to be an abrogative threat to liberty, one that erodes individuals' capacity to repel domination and exposing them to the power of others—not least to an arbitrary and inactive neoliberal state that has failed to promote sufficient health equity over recent years.

Conclusion

In his book *Development as Freedom*, Indian economist Amartya Sen (1999) argues that the success of social and spatial development strategies must be measured not in terms of Gross Domestic Product (GDP) or rising standards of living but instead on the extent to which human freedom is enhanced. Poverty should not be construed only in terms of the absence of wealth and income but should include in addition the extent to which an individual is free to make and realize particular choices—that is, to live the life they have reason to value. Freedom ought to be both the intended outcome of development and the principal means through which development is achieved. Freedom is good in and of itself; it is also good because it leads to human self-actualization, increases social effectiveness, spurs innovation, and creates growth. For Sen, the expansion of five particular freedoms is central to development:

political freedoms, economic facilities, social opportunities, transparency guarantees, and protective security. It is the role of human rights law to safeguard these freedoms, enable people to make choices and acquire capabilities, and catalyze development.

However, by pursuing an ideal of freedom as non-interference, and by delegitimising the potential for the democratic state to intervene proactively to promote the common good, the neoliberal project has made the UK both a less equal and less free country. One where the rich and powerful have been enabled to exploit, manipulate, and profit from the rest, whilst we are all less secure against the threat of emergency. If the UK is to meaningfully *build back better* it will be imperative that the state no longer treats widening inequality with indifference or invests in the demonstrable false assumption that what the market breaks the market fixes. The state need not be neutral towards the inequalities thrown up by capitalist markets. Freedom does not demand inattention and inaction. Indeed, freedom as non-domination requires instead that the state becomes, again, a democratic mechanism for equalising the standing between citizens in society, enabling them to interact on a standing of shared freedom. This will require a rediscovery and reinforcement of the UK's social democratic foundations, developing renewed public institutions necessary to develop the level of shared health, wealth, and security necessary for each individual to look others in the eye as a free and equal citizen.

References

Bambra, C., Riordan, R., Ford, J., & Matthews, F. (2020). The COVID-19 pandemic and health inequalities. *Journal of Epidemiology and Community Health, 74*(11), 964–968.

Beveridge, F. (2020). Inequality in the Face of COVID-19: How do we build back stronger in the Liverpool city region? *University of Liverpool Heseltine Institute Policy Brief*, 27.

Chancel, L., Piketty, T., & Saez, E. (Eds.) (2022). *World inequality report 2022.* Harvard University Press.

Hanlon, P. (2015). Unhealthy glasgow: A case for ecological public health? *Public Health, 129*(10), 1353–1360.

Marmot, M. (2010). *Fair society, healthy lives: Strategic review of health inequalities in England post 2010.* Marmot Review.

Marmot, M., et al. (2020). *Health equity in England: The Marmot review 10 years on.* Institute of Health Equity.

McCann, P. (2016). *The UK regional-national economic problem: Geography, globalisation and governance.* Routledge.

McCann, P. (2020). Perceptions of regional inequality and the geography of discontent: Insights from the UK. *Regional Studies, 54*(2), 256–267.

McCann, P., Ortega-Argilés, R., & Yuan, P.-Y. (2022). The Covid-19 shock in European regions. *Regional Studies, 56*(7), 1142–1160.

Nozick, R. (1974). *Anarchy, state, and utopia.* Blackwell.

Pettit, P. (1996). Freedom as anti-power. *Ethics, 106*(3), 576–604.

Pettit, P. (1997). *Republicanism: A theory of freedom and government.* Oxford University Press.

Pettit, P. (2007). A republican right to basic income? *Basic Income Studies, 2*(2), 1–8.

Pettit, P. (2010). Civic republican theory. In J. L. Martí & P. Pettit (Eds.), *A political philosophy in public life: Civic republicanism in Zapatero's Spain.* Princeton University Press.

Pettit, P. (2012). *On the people's terms: A republican theory and model of democracy.* Cambridge University Press.

Piketty, T. (2020). *Capital and ideology.* Harvard University Press.

Schofield, J., Leelarathna, L., & Thabit, H. (2020). COVID-19: Impact of and on diabetes. *Diabetes Therapy, 11*(7), 1429–1435.

Sen, A. (1999). *Development as freedom.* Knopf.

Singer, M. (2009). *Introduction to syndemics: A critical systems approach to public and community health.* John Wiley & Sons.

Smith, N. (1984). *Uneven development: Nature. Capital, and the production of space.* Blackwell.

Taylor-Robinson, D., Whitehead, M., & Barr, B. (2014). Great leap backwards. *British Medical Journal, 349*, g7350.

UK2070. (2020). *Make no little plans: Acting at scale for a fairer and stronger future.* UK2070 Commission.

Wang, B., Li, R., Lu, Z., & Huang, Y. (2020). Does comorbidity increase the risk of patients with COVID-19: Evidence from meta-analysis. *Aging, 12*(7), 6049.

Whitehead, M., McInroy, N., & Bambra, C., et al. (2014). *Due North report of the inquiry on health equity in the North.* University of Liverpool and the Centre for Economic Strategies.

Whitehead, M., Taylor-Robinson, D., & Barr, B. (2014). Great leap backwards. *British Medical Journal, 349*. https://doi.org/10.1136/bmj.g7350

Wilkinson, R., & Pickett, K. (2010). *The spirit level: Why equality is better for everyone.* Penguin.

Wilkinson, R., & Pickett, K. (2020). *The inner level: How more equal societies reduce stress, restore sanity and improve everyone's well-being.* Penguin.

CHAPTER 8

Reclaiming Freedom: Placing Republican Thought in the Service of 'build back better'

Abstract In this concluding chapter, we restate the key findings of our analysis and clarify why the COVID-19 pandemic must—morally and practically—represent a breaking point away from neoliberalism. We pre-emptively warn against a regenerated, post-pandemic neoliberalism (neoliberalism redux), offering instead a constructive neorepublican alternative that directly challenges dominant assumptions about the meaning of liberty, the potential of the state, the roles and responsibilities of the citizen, and the permissibility of gross socioeconomic inequality. This distinctly antineoliberal alternative, we argue, offers a philosophical foundation from which to reimagine a model of social democracy for the twenty-first century, promoting individual liberty through the maintenance of a proactive and protective democratic state.

Keywords Anti-neoliberalism · Neo-republicanism · Build back better · Social democracy · Freedom as non-domination · Equality of opportunity · c21st states

© The Author(s), under exclusive license to Springer Nature Switzerland AG 2022
M. Boyle et al., *COVID-19 and the Case Against Neoliberalism*, https://doi.org/10.1007/978-3-031-18935-7_8

INTRODUCTION

At the time of writing, the global COVID-19 pandemic remains far from over. On 4 May 2022, the Director-General of the World Health Organisation, Tedros Adhanom Ghebreyesus cautioned that, although globally reported cases and deaths from COVID-19 are declining, the emergence of new variants, uneven vaccination rates, slow or non-existent testing, and genetic sequencing, and unequal access to antiviral treatments mean that the world still faces a significant threat from the virus: "We're playing with a fire that continues to burn us".

That SARS-CoV-2 has dealt such a fateful impact across the globe—particularly when compared to the much more limited SARS-CoV-1 outbreak that occurred between 2002 and 2004—should be understood as a global failure. Scientific research may determine that there was something particular about SARS-CoV-2, its biology and virology, that meant a global pandemic of a significant scale was always likely, if not to some degree inevitable. Indeed, despite all medical and technological development, human beings will always remain essentially fragile and vulnerable creatures in the face of emerging and re-emerging communicable diseases. Nevertheless, the precise course, trajectory, and severity of the COVID-19 pandemic have also been a product of politics. There is no such thing as an entirely natural disaster, with the scale and scope of the crisis influenced by inherited political logics and legacies, and the choices, actions, and (in)decisions of global governments.

This book has sought to reveal, explain, and critique the political nature of the pandemic, arguing that political ideas, and policies, inform the vulnerability of different states to crisis. How governments coordinate and utilise national resources, when interventions are or are not deployed, how narratives are constructed: these matter, and will continue to matter, as societies seek to recover and rebuild resilience in the coming years.

The story of the pandemic in the UK has been offered in these pages as illustrative or emblematic, though not necessarily paradigmatic, of the global political failure to contain and attenuate the impact of COVID-19 on lives and livelihoods. Our claim is not that the UK was the *worst* performer globally, or that it was somehow *uniquely* vulnerable to the pandemic threat. Instead, we want to suggest that the UK perhaps *typifies* the political (and philosophical) failings that have hindered humanity's capacity to limit the spread of COVID-19.

We therefore offer a nuanced analysis of the UK's pandemic performance. One that, as a consequence of the rapid nature with which the evidence has been reviewed, also remains partial and incomplete. It would be naïve and simplistic to argue that the UK has not, at various points, responded appropriately and effectively to the pandemic. Indeed, where the UK has sufficiently unlocked the full potential of the state, for example with its early vaccine rollout, it has been truly world leading. However, performance has been erratic to say the least, with a response that has also often been hesitant, negligent, and self-defeating.

The central argument of this book is that this erratic performance can be someway explained by studying the underlying political philosophical commitment, held by the Johnson government, to neoliberal ideas and approaches to thinking about freedom, the state, the citizen, and inequality. Where the state has indulged these neoliberal instincts, either implicitly or explicitly, it has failed to sufficiently control the pandemic or minimise its impacts, and instead feigned impotence. Hindered by a commitment to the logic of neoliberalism, the British state has also been constrained by the long-term legacies of four decades of neoliberal policymaking, which have served to significantly erode state capacity and undermine the resilience of people, communities, and economies to crisis.

With public inquiry processes now gathering momentum across the globe, not least in the UK itself, what lessons should be learned from this cautionary tale, and how can these lessons help us to break out of the vicious cycle of perpetual crisis that we find ourselves in?

In this concluding chapter, we restate the key findings of our analysis and clarify why the COVID-19 pandemic must—morally and practically— represent a breaking point away from neoliberalism. We pre-emptively warn against a regenerated, post-pandemic neoliberalism (neoliberalism redux), offering instead a constructive neorepublican alternative that directly challenges dominant assumptions about the meaning of liberty, the potential of the state, the roles and responsibilities of the citizen, and the permissibility of gross socioeconomic inequality. This distinctly *antineoliberal* alternative, we argue, offers a philosophical foundation from which to reimagine social democracy for the twenty-first century, promoting individual liberty *through* the maintenance of a proactive and protective democratic state.

LIVING WITH COVID-19 AND NEOLIBERALISM REDUX

In spite of dire predictions and apocalyptic forecasts, neoliberalism has shown itself to be resilient and tenacious. According to David Harvey, neoliberalism's record of securing economic growth has been 'dismal', comparing unfavourably to Keynesianism in its prime. However, it has been hugely successful in temporarily staving off the falling rate of profit and crises in capital accumulation that prevailed in the mid-1970s. In so doing, its main achievements have been 'redistributive rather than generative' (Harvey, 2005, p. 153). For Harvey, neoliberalism is best conceived of as a political project designed to restore class power by returning the division of the national product between competing class fractions back to pre-Keynesian levels. This has been managed through the introduction of new forms of 'accumulation by dispossession', including the privatisation and commodification of virtually everything everywhere, financialization, the management and manipulation of crises, and state redistributions.

This book is intended as a contribution to literature on the dialectic between the reassertion of neoliberal institutions globally in the post-COVID-19 era and the active and contingent making and remaking of concrete neoliberalisations in specific countries. Informed by Peck, Theodore and Brenner's theorisation of disaster capitalism and post-crisis neoliberalism redux and alert to the variegated geographies of and the importance of place specific politico-institutional formations in post-COVID-19 regulatory experimentation, we construe the UKs post-crash embrace of deepened neoliberalism as comprising an ongoing series of provisional, contested and contingent regulatory redesigns. Our thesis is that to view any apparent continuity as a simple reset after a shock or a blip is to err; instead, any embrace of neoliberalism redux must be viewed as an active, historically novel, contested and ultimately vulnerable reinvention and reimagining.

A key question we seek to investigate is to what extent these parameters have been challenged by the current pandemic and its attendant cascading crises. To address this, we now turn our attention to the role of discursive and symbolic fiction in sustaining our everyday reality.

The capacity of neoliberalism to secure a social licence has rested in no small way on its formidable power to manufacture consent. Against the backdrop of the expansion of capitalism after the fall of state socialism and the intensification of neoliberal economic policies, Jacques Ranciere (1995, 1999) claims that liberal market democracies have entered into a phase of illiberal 'post-democracy'. "To the extent that state authority is increasingly less able to constrain corporate power, politics matter less" (Dean, 2009, 11), while the consensus-based approach of deliberative democracy and the celebration of the individualised neoliberal subject have combined to diminish 'the political'. For Ranciere 'politics' (sometimes referred to as the 'police') is "the art of suppressing the political" (Ranciere, 1995, 11), while 'the political' is an extremely determined activity antagonistic to policing" (Ranciere, 1999, 29). The public sphere is "a sphere of encounters and conflicts between the two opposed logics of police and politics [and thus the] spontaneous practices of any government tend to shrink this public sphere" by 'disavowing' the political (Ranciere, 2006, 55). Government is oligarchic and politics only occurs in fleeting moments of 'disagreement' (Ranciere, 1999), a point of articulation outside the police order, but which aims at transforming it.

Theorists of the post-political generally agree that the current constellation more forcefully disavows the political in that "[p]roper political questions always involve decisions that require making a choice between conflicting alternatives" (Mouffe, 2013, 3). Under these conditions, "adversarial politics (of the left/right variety or of radically divergent struggles over imagining and naming different socio-environmental futures, for example) are considered hopelessly out of date" and debate and disagreement operate within "an overall model of elite consensus and agreement" (Swyngedouw, 2009, 610). Mouffe (2000, 2005, 2013) sees a way out of this impasse through a reformation of the institutions of liberal democracy to better enable 'agonistic' politics of a pluralist nature to flourish. Žižek's (1999, 236) concern, however, is that the current formation of "post-modern post-politics… no longer merely 'represses' the political, trying to contain it and pacify the 'returns of the repressed', but much more effectively 'forecloses' it". Politics is, thus, foreclosed he argues because "a properly political act would necessarily entail the repoliticization of the economy". With the basic rules set in advance, technocratic management solutions will always be put forward for the situation 'as it stands'. This forecloses the art of the impossible, which is the very ground for politics (Žižek, 1999, 237).

In February 2022, the UK government published its *Living With Covid-19* strategy, setting out the country's forward approach to a now endemic and enduring virus, albeit one that appears less dangerous thanks to a successful vaccination campaign that has provided much of the population with a significant (though incomplete) level of protection from its worst effects. Written in dry, technocratic language, rather than the emotive political vocabulary of liberty, the document nonetheless continues to reflect the neoliberal ideas and instincts that have been central to the UK's pandemic response, and to this book.

With emergency restrictions no longer deemed necessary, the roles and responsibilities of the state to combat COVID-19 have been minimised further. The state now aims to treat COVID-19 "like other respiratory illnesses" (HM Government, 2022, 7); relying, in future, on vaccines to bring down hospitalisations and deaths, and sufficient health service capacity to cope with future COVID-19 patients as they arise, rather than mandated social distancing. The government has ended the provision of free testing kits to the majority of the general public, promoting instead the creation of private markets to maintain testing capacity and coverage. Routine contact tracing has also ended, along with the legal requirement to self-isolate following a positive test (ibid., 16–19). Meanwhile, the document emphasises the perceived "opportunities", created as a result of the pandemic, to increase investment in the UK's life sciences sector and promote the UK economy (ibid., 38).

This reflects the neoliberal instinct, discussed in Chapter 5, to minimise direct state intervention whenever and wherever possible and to prioritise, instead, utilising the power of the state to create, maintain, and expand markets. If only a minimal state can be justified, as neoliberals assume, then we can understand why the UK government would be keen to cast aside any responsibility for proactive health protection interventions, such as the maintenance of a mass test and trace system. Even if such interventions may still be valuable for monitoring the continuing trajectory and evolution of the virus, they are likely to be viewed by neoliberals as an unjustifiable overreach of government interference in the lives of individuals, and an intolerable burden on 'the tax payer'. Indeed, the government argues explicitly that the £15.7 billion spent on test, trace, and isolation in the UK during the 2020–2021 financial year is a figure that can no longer be justified (HM Government, 2022, 17–18).

As the state has withdrawn, citizens are now expected to take greater personal responsibility for the collective health of the nation. The emphasis now from the UK government is on "encouraging safer behaviours through public health advice" (HM Government, 2022, 8). Similarly, businesses will no longer be mandated to explicitly consider

COVID-19 in their risk assessments. Instead, the government intends to "empower businesses to take responsibility for implementing mitigations that are appropriate for their circumstances" (ibid., 20). This echoes the neoliberal model of citizenship discussed in Chapter 6, which valorises personal responsibility over collective democracy. However, taking personal responsibility, and making responsible decisions, in the middle of a global pandemic is more difficult when you can no longer easily determine whether you pose a risk, or are at risk, from COVID-19 thanks to a free and accessible test, trace, and isolation system. Moreover, as the government has removed legal restrictions it has also ended self-isolation support payments, national funding for practical support, and other measures such as the medicine delivery service which had been in place to help the most vulnerable through the pandemic. COVID-19 provisions within Statutory Sick Pay and Employment and Support Allowance regulations have also been withdrawn, meaning that people with COVID-19 may no longer be eligible for financial support if they are too ill to work (ibid., 17). Compelled by the necessity to keep working, and keep businesses open, citizens have little tangible power to do the right thing and self-isolate if they suspect they have COVID, enabling the virus to continue circulating—and mutating—within the community.

This is likely to further exacerbate the inequalities that have been exploited by the pandemic to date, exposing the most vulnerable and most disadvantaged to the most risk as the virus continues to evolve and cause serious harm (albeit at a less severe scale than that seen in 2020 and 2021). As outlined in this chapter, the corrosive effect that neoliberal insouciance towards inequality has had on the UK's resilience to crisis has been starkly highlighted by the pandemic. Nevertheless, where the *Living with Covid* strategy recognises the need to now redress health inequalities, detail on how this will actually be achieved is vague, if not perfunctory. The UK government appears to have failed to learn the lesson presented by COVID-19, that there is a pragmatic as well as moral reason to disrupt the vicious cycle that exists between widening socioeconomic inequality and poor health outcomes.

All this suggests that the UK Government continues to be constrained, implicitly and explicitly, by the norms and assumptions of neoliberal thought, and in particular the idea that the cause of individual freedom is best served by minimising state interference in the lives of citizens, and in the function of the economy, as much as possible. As shown throughout this book, the destructive logic and legacies of neoliberalism stem from a particular understanding of liberty, strictly conceptualised as non-interference. It is this conceptualisation of freedom that underpins how neoliberals think about the state, citizen, and inequality; and it is this conceptualisation of freedom, and its valorisation, that has undermined the UK's resilience, preparedness, and capacity for effective crisis response. Placing the right of individuals to exercise their economic sovereignty as paramount, and seeking to insulate these individuals and the markets they operate in from interference or constraint by the state, neoliberalism presents policymakers with a limited choice architecture. However, this choice architecture cannot be transformed without first reclaiming the politically valuable language of freedom, and challenging how it is understood in political discourse.

Despite initial calls that COVID-19 would represent a watershed moment from which the UK, and the world, would 'build back better', the *Living With Covid* strategy could be read as a first step towards neoliberalism redux, a continuation and consolidation of neoliberal ideas and instincts that will now inform post-pandemic recovery and long-term renewal. Not only does neoliberalism redux risk perpetuating widening inequality, deepening poverty, and intensifying precarity, it also risks further eroding the capacity of individuals, communities, and economies to respond effectively to the mounting crises facing society in the twenty-first century.

Indeed, we have lurched from a public health crisis and into a cost of living crisis, driven by global inflation, energy insecurity, the Russian invasion of Ukraine, and a backlog of disruption to international supply chains caused by the pandemic (see, for example, IfG, 2022). With wages unable to keep up with spiralling bills, many in the UK are faced with extreme hardship and poverty. Analysis by the National Institute of Economic and Social Research suggests that consumer price index inflation to average 7.8 per cent in 2022, whilst real incomes will decline by 2.4 per cent. For the 2022–2023 financial year NIESR estimate that 1.5 million households will face food and energy bills that outstrip their disposable income. Meanwhile, the Resolution Foundation estimates that this wages and bills crisis will see a further 1.3 million people, including 500,000 children, fall into absolute poverty over the same period (Resolution Foundation, 2022).

However, the UK government appears to be sticking to their neoliberal playbook of delay, hesitancy, and reticence; unwilling to intervene significantly and directly in the economy. The government has offered some relief, mostly through tax cuts, but has so far failed to introduce targeted interventions to help people sufficiently meet the spiralling cost of living (see, for example, HM Treasury, 2022). In particular, the government has appeared reluctant to significantly raise taxes on the most wealthy, including via a windfall tax on the record profits of oil and gas companies, with Boris Johnson arguing that this "clobbers the very businesses that we need to invest in energy to bring the prices down for people across this country" (Hansard, 27 April 2022, col 755). This state inaction, combined with a preference for market-based solutions, suggests a continuation of orthodox neoliberal policymaking instincts that have been unaltered by the potentially transformative experience of the COVID-19 pandemic.

This unwillingness to engage in coordinated, proactive, and disruptive state intervention to ward off looming crises also raises significant doubts about the UK's current capacity to respond sufficiently to the truly existential crisis of our times, an accelerating climate and ecological emergency. As the Intergovernmental Panel on Climate Change (IPCC, 2022) has made clear, a rapid, deep, and systemic transition away from greenhouse gas emissions is urgently needed to ensure that median global warming does not exceed 1.5 degrees centigrade above pre-industrial temperatures. However, the necessary decarbonisation of the ways we collectively live, work, and get around can only be driven by ambitious state intervention. Individuals and businesses alone simply do not have the means, or incentives, to drive this change wholly and sufficiently from the bottom up. Whilst the UK government has set out ambitious climate targets, enshrining in law that emissions must be cut by at least 78% by 2035, there is still insufficient evidence that the necessary scale and scope of national transformation is being actively delivered by the government. In 2021, the UK's Climate Change Committee (CCC) reported that the delivery of climate change mitigation and adaptation policy remained too slow, with inaction moving the UK further off course to meet its climate targets. More effective and proactive policies are now required at greater pace if we are to stay on track. However, we may reasonably fear that an entrenched neoliberal presumption against state intervention is unlikely to support such an approach.

The neoliberal world appears trapped in a vicious cycle of near-perpetual crisis; one that is of its own making. A system that cultivates (or, at the very least, accepts) a context of perpetual crisis, that promotes state impotence in the face of these crises, and that exposes millions of people to precarity, poverty, and inequality would, in the words of political philosopher John Rawls, be considered to impose excessive "strains of commitment" on the majority of citizens (2001, 104; see also Lefkowitz, 2014, 813–816). Why should we, as individuals, reasonably accept and affirm a political and economic status quo that consistently fails to function in a way that promotes and protects our shared interests as citizens? A decisive break with the neoliberal order is now required.

Neorepublicanism and Twenty-First-Century Social Democracy

It is one thing to ask whether COVID-19 *has* disrupted the 'distribution of the sensible' and traumatised the discourses and the symbolic fictions upon which the staging of neoliberal society depends. It is quite another to ask, *could* the pandemic serve as a potential turning point in political history, a moment through which to glimpse the possibilities of a new world, and build bridges to a different future (see, for example, Painter, 2020; Roy, 2020; etc.). It is our view that this is indeed a moment of great upheaval and neoliberalism is indeed coming close to exhausting its capacity to garner a social licence. But any historical pivot will be impossible to achieve unless we systematically and deliberately break with the ideas and instincts of neoliberalism, cultivating an alternative public political philosophy that challenges neoliberal assumptions about freedom, the state, the citizen, and the permissibility of widening inequality.

This book has identified the seeds of such an alternative, locating them within the neorepublican tradition of political theory. Our claim here is modest. We do not necessarily hold that neorepublicanism offers the only, or even the best, possible alternative to neoliberalism. Our claim instead is that it offers one *plausible* and, we believe, achievable alternative.

As we have shown over the preceding chapters, neorepublican theory offers a direct counterpoint to neoliberalism; one that remains similarly rooted in a preeminent concern for the political value of individual liberty. In this respect, we suggest, neorepublicanism offers a potentially crucial foundation from which to develop an *antineoliberal* politics for the twenty-first century.

In contrast to neoliberal conceptions of freedom, republicans define liberty not as non-interference, but non-domination. The most influential contemporary republican political theorist, Philip Pettit, defines such domination as the capacity, exercised or unexercised, for one agent to wield power arbitrarily over another, at will and with impunity (1997, 52–55). On this definition, one can be made unfree even when no actual interference has taken place; it is the *capacity*, the tangible potential, for interference that is enough to undermine one's free status. Moreover, the republican conceptualisation of freedom also suggests that not all interference is deleterious of individual liberty. Non-arbitrary interference, such as that associated with the free and fair rule of law, is not understood to pose a threat to liberty so long as it is forced to function in the common interest and not the discretionary whim of a particular agent (ibid., 65, 174, 183–186). Indeed, to the extent that non-arbitrary laws or interventions serve to insulate and insure individuals against potential sources of domination in society, such interference can be seen to, in fact, *constitute* one's freedom, by providing effective communal immunity against domination (Pettit, 2002, 347).

For republicans, the state therefore does not essentially or necessarily pose a threat to individual freedom. Instead it is seen as a potential mechanism through which individuals can create, maintain, and guarantee the particular political and social conditions that promote and facilitate freedom. After all, "it is only possible to be free in a free state" (Skinner, 2012, 60). For this reason, republicans are less sceptical of state intervention and activism. So long as it is constitutionally designed to prevent the partial, arbitrary exercise of power—for example, through the rule of law, separation of powers, and democratic checks on public decision-making (Pettit, 1997, 171–205)—republicans are entirely comfortable with granting the state "a considerable range of responsibilities" (ibid., 150) across society and the economy. In contrast to the neoliberal ideal of the minimal state, then, neorepublicans may endorse a much more expansive state, one which acts as "an agency that moulds and shapes society" (Pettit, 2010, 39).

To reiterate, however, this does not mean that republicans are naïve to the potential threat that state power could pose to freedom. Should governments have the capacity to act *arbitrarily* in the lives of citizens, without required reference to their ideas and interests—as under a dictatorship—then republicans would certainly condemn such a state as insufficiently republican and incompatible with liberty. But rather than rejecting state intervention out of hand as abrogative of individual freedom, republicans instead argue for enhanced democratic control of the state—via the creation and maintenance of opportunities for vigilant and actively contestatory citizenship—in order to both counter the threat of domination by the state and authorise legitimate forms proactive state intervention that pursues the common good (Pettit, 1997, 183–185). In contrast to the denuded model of citizenship cultivated by neoliberalism, neorepublicanism encourages citizens to take ownership of the state as a machine for solidaristic, collective self-government. Citizenship is not just a status, but a way of life whereby individuals work both with and against the state in order to guarantee their freedom and democratically discover how best to promote their shared interests.

As Pettit, states, "not only will republicans tend to be less sceptical in regard to state action; they will also be more radical in relation to social policy...They will take a more radical view of the ills that government is called upon to rectify" (Pettit, 1997, 149). Chief among these ills will be the causes and consequences of inequalities between citizens. Freedom as non-domination demands "intersubjective equality" (ibid., 64), whereby citizens can relate to each other effectively as equals. This requires a suitably republican state to proactively minimise socioeconomic inequalities, and prevent them from translating into the kinds of intersubjective power imbalances that promote domination (ibid., 118). Inequality is therefore not something to be tolerated in order to promote freedom, it is something to combat in order to promote freedom. As such, neorepublicans are more likely to both inherently value and proactively pursue greater equality between citizens than their neoliberal counterparts.

From this neorepublican vantage point we can more clearly see the political and philosophical contingency of the UK government's response to the COVID-19, and the extent to which the potential for effective and timely intervention was constrained by adherence to neoliberal logics, and the longer-term legacies of historical neoliberal policymaking. Neorepublicanism emphasises how, whilst still maintaining a paramount focus on the value of individual liberty, the state could have legitimately responded to the pandemic threat in a harder, faster, and more coordinated way, in line with international best practice. Moreover, this vantage point emphasises the needlessness with which the British state has eroded the public realm over recent decades, undermining the resilience of people, communities, and the economy in the name of freedom. For republicans the cause of freedom is, instead, best served through an expansive state, a vigilant citizenry, and the cultivation of a more equal society: factors that may have strengthened the UK's resilience to COVID-19 had they not been critically damaged by decades of neoliberal policymaking.

With these lessons learned, how might neorepublican ideas now inform the project of post-pandemic recovery and renewal, as states such as the UK look to 'build back better'?

Republicanism is a tradition of political thought that tends to focus more on constitutional design than promoting particular, pre-determined, and universally ideal, political outcomes. It emphasises the creation and maintenance of appropriate institutions to prevent domination, both by the state and other powerful agents in society, however, how the ideal of freedom as non-domination is best pursued within a suitably republican state is open to interpretation by the citizens of that time and place. Republicanism, in this respect, offers an open-ended process of continual deliberation and discovery in order to maximise our shared freedom, and our protection from domination. As Pettit explains: "To endorse republican freedom is not to accept a ready-made ideal that can be applied in a mechanical way, now to this group, now to that. It is to embrace an open-ended ideal that gains new substance and relevance as it is interpreted in the progressively changing and clarifying perspectives of a living society" (Pettit, 1997, 147).

For this reason, there are multiple possible interpretations of republican ideas, and republican political programmes, that could be offered in the service of the post-pandemic, build back better project. The history of the republican tradition suggests that a spectrum of interpretations, ranging from the conservative to the radical (see, for example, Leipold et al., 2020), is possible. Nevertheless, our initial, and transitional, recommendation here is for neorepublicans to promote a rediscovery and reimagination of social democracy.

Social democracy describes a particular kind of relationship between the state, the market, and society whereby democratic collective action extends "the principles of freedom and equality valued by democrats in the political sphere to the organization of the economy and society, chiefly by opposing the inequality and oppression created by laissez-faire capitalism". Typically, this is achieved by ensuring that the market is embedded within, and guided by, a state-led framework of regulation and interventionist economic policy to help ensure it functions to support the public good. Universalist systems for welfare and social insurance, as well as essential public services, are established and maintained by the state to narrow inequalities and improve quality of life. Progressive taxation, and the public investment it affords, is viewed as conducive to progress and development. And this is all mediated, and legitimised, through the nurturing of a peaceful, open-ended democratic culture through which society and the economy can be continuously improved (ibid.).

A "post-war consensus" that formed around a broadly social democratic vision of the state provided the foundation for the political, economic, and institutional model we have in Britain today. Notably this period included the creation of the welfare state (including the National Health Service), as well as the development of government capacity to intervene actively in the economy, for example through counter-cyclical fiscal policy, the nationalisation of strategic industries, collective bargaining with labour unions, and progressive levels of taxation. However, in calling for a reimagination and rediscovery of the UK's social democratic foundations we do not intend necessarily to make a nostalgic argument that yearns for a return to some perceived "golden age" between 1945 and 1975. Instead we argue that, to build back better from the pandemic, the state must recapture the spirit and the purpose of mid-century social democracy, reinterpret how social democratic ideas can be relevant in the context of the twenty-first century, and then redesign the social democratic institutional frameworks that underpin our politico-economic system.

Philip Pettit has already established how neorepublican ideas can underpin a "broadly social democratic agenda" (Pettit, 2010, 49, 54–58). Nevertheless, this agenda will need to be re-evaluated, reinterpreted, and regenerated in the context of post-pandemic destruction, neoliberal perma-crisis, and, in the UK especially, the corrosive effects of neoliberal hegemony on pre-existing foundations of social democracy.

A full account of a neorepublican, social democratic political programme for post-pandemic recovery, renewal, and resilience building may be beyond the limits of this short book. Nevertheless, we offer here an initial sketch of this model, with an emphasis on two key recommendations. To meet the needs of the twenty-first century, neorepublican social democracy must:

(i) renew the active democratic role of the citizen, in order to,
(ii) rebuild the capacity of the state to legitimately redress inequality, combat precarity, and proactively avert (and effectively mitigate) crises.

To renew the active democratic role of the citizen, we must cultivate meaningful constitutional and institutional opportunities for vigilant contestation. Above and beyond the often distant, and elitist, electoral politics of Westminster, we must experiment with forms of participatory and deliberative models of democracy, actively encouraging opportunities for citizens to invigilate the decisions of elected politicians and their officials, and to complement abstract bureaucratic governance with the real ideas, hopes, and aspirations of those people the state is designed to serve. Mechanisms such as citizens assemblies and other forms of meaningful public consultation, idea generation, and collaborative problem solving—should be formalised and normalised throughout policymaking and service design processes to increase the quality and legitimacy of the decisions and actions taken by public organisations. In this way, the neoliberal parody of the state as an impersonal, impassive, and ineffective bureaucracy can be shattered, and instead the development of the state can become a genuine, shared, and open-ended enterprise with citizens to realise the common good.

The economy too should be brought further into the purview of democratic oversight, scrutiny, and influence. The belief that people have a right to vote for political parties and shape the direction of governments is widely accepted. What is less accepted is that they also have a right to participate in the design of the economy as a whole: how and what to tax, where investment is to go, what is to be subsidised, workers' rights, regulatory standards and restrictions and so on? Older traditions of economic democracy based upon ideas of public ownership and the collective bargaining of mass-member labour unions should be augmented with three new critical interlocking pillars: individual economic rights, diverse forms of democratic collective ownership and control of companies, and greater public participation in economic decision-making (Cumbers, 2020).

By embracing a more active role for citizens to ensure that political and economic decisions track the interests of those they affect, we can deliver an antidote to the denuded and infantilised public sphere propagated by neoliberalism. A vibrant public square must be nurtured alongside an invigorated culture of debate and futurity speech—that is, the capacity to imagine different, hopeful, and aspirational, futures. In contrast to the neoliberal axiom that there is no alternative, we must acknowledge that there is always an alternative, and that citizens have a right and capacity to demand it. Indeed, democratic politics should always be a continuous and iterative process of discovering and realising the needs, and ambitions, and ideas of citizens as these evolve over time.

Citizens must be able to contribute meaningfully and actively to the design and development of the future, particularly in the context of rapid disruption to the status quo as a result of the lasting impacts of the pandemic, the advancement of new technologies, and the mounting imperative to address the climate emergency. To rebuild the trust in the social contract that has been so critically eroded by four decades of neoliberalism, people must now be given a renewed sense of ownership in the political and economic life of the society in which they live. They must be the chief architects of any renewed social democratic state, and the authors of what building back better really means.

Opportunities for vigilant, contestatory democracy, and the cultivation of a vibrant culture of public futurity speech, will be critical if we are to then safely renew the roles and responsibilities of the state as we build back better from the pandemic. We need no longer view the legitimate role of the democratic state merely as a guarantor of market functions, but instead as the means by which we collectively shape the world to support the public good. Challenging neoliberal assumptions about the legitimate role of the state in this way will be necessary if we are to proactively arrest and reverse the widening, corrosive inequalities in society. It will be necessary to coordinate and manage an effective recovery from the pandemic. And it will be necessary as we look to increase our resilience and proactively respond to future crises, not least the accelerating climate emergency.

Reclaiming the social democratic culture and capacity of the British state in this way will require the rebuilding of a public realm decimated by four decades of neoliberalism, and in particular, a decade of austerity. The minimal, austere state cultivated over multiple decades in adherence to neoliberal ideology has been shown to be slow, dysfunctional, and ill-prepared for crisis.

In the first instance, this means reversing public spending cuts to provide state agencies with the latitude and the resources necessary to provide high-quality and readily accessible frontline services and social infrastructure. From social housing to public transport, public health to social services, children's centres, libraries, and public parks; these are the services that people and communities need to survive, thrive, and reliably resist domination and exploitation by powerful economic and social agents. Rebuilding the public realm also means regenerating central government's institutional capacity to deliver vital public services, not least health, education, and social insurance, in a way that provides a solid foundation of welfare to all citizens as a right. This is critical for the enjoyment of freedom as non-domination. Indeed, Pettit has argued that republican liberty demands "a more or less constitutional guarantee of welfare provision, with some independent, depoliticized means of determining levels of provision" (Pettit, 1997, 162). Reconstructing the social safety net will help to reduce intersubjective inequalities of all kinds, and provide a shared basis of security for all citizens. Such a social safety net, constructed as a universal public good, will be more critical than ever in an era of disruption and transformation as society emerges from the pandemic.

The state must also regain its legitimate capacity to intervene confidently in the economy. The state must be seen as a mechanism through which democratic citizens can influence and coordinate the economy to ensure it serves the common interests of all citizens rather than the partial interests of the powerful. This does not necessarily mean the whole economy should be completely controlled by central government, but that the state—through regulation, investment, and the expansion of public ownership where appropriate—recognises its ability to guide the economy and influence its outcomes, rather than allowing unfettered capitalism to continue generating vast inequality, poverty, and environmental collapse.

In order for this to happen, though, the state must also articulate a renewed, positive case for taxation. Contrary to neoliberal fears that taxation represents an unjustifiable infringement on the economic independence of individuals, tax should not be thought of as a form of enforced charity or 'robbing the rich to give to the poor'. Instead, it should be seen as emblematic of our shared commitment to living in a free and fair society. Indeed, it is through taxation that we can together ensure we live in a secure, stable, and functioning democracy that enables everyone to enjoy a decent quality of life as a right; a quality of life that could not be achieved by individuals working in isolation. Coercive redistribution may also be necessary to limit the dominating power of extraordinary, concentrated wealth, and the potential this creates for disproportionate influence over the economic, social, and political life of the community. Taxation is therefore not a burden to be tolerated or an all-things-considered permissible infringement on our liberty for the greater good; it is fundamentally constitutive of our intersubjective status as free, independent, and equal citizens in a society. A society where we each have the ability to command the resources of our shared community to protect and respect this status through the activities of the state.

However, building back better will require more than simply reversing the damage of neoliberalism to the public realm and public discourse, it will also require recapturing the spirit of social democracy, to reimagine the potential of the state as a positive force for human development in the context of the twenty-first century and beyond.

Taking inspiration from the example of the New Zealand government's recent wellbeing budgets, this should mean moving beyond thinking about the state as just a guarantor of 'safety net' welfare, but also as a means to ensure that the ways we live and work together actively promote the shared wellbeing of all citizens in the first place. Rather than outsourcing human development to the exigencies of the free market, a neorepublican, social democratic wellbeing state should prioritise and pursue human flourishing in the broadest sense, by maintaining the legal, social, political, economic, and environmental conditions necessary to achieve this. This means that the state should work proactively to support the health, wealth, and wellbeing of all citizens, communities, and the natural environment, protecting the fundamental bases that enable human life to thrive. Without this, disadvantaged groups will continue to face the threat of domination by those who are able to control critical resources necessary not only for survival, but for a good quality of life.

This would require new regulations, institutions, and interventions to ensure society and the economy respect the quality and value of all human life, as well as the limits of our natural environment (e.g. Raworth, 2017). These could include the introduction of real living wages and living hours regulations to improve the quality of working life; the introduction of a Universal Basic Income and Universal Basic Services to provide everyone with a secure foundation of material resources; and a coordinated Green New Deal (Klein, 2020) to build the infrastructure and support mechanisms for a fair, just, and rapid transition to a sustainable economy (see also, Barry, 2021). The state must, in other words, become an effective mechanism through which we ensure the world around us supports the best possible life, and the best possible future, free of domination for all; *predistributing* a shared basis of wellbeing to prevent unjust inequalities emerging in the first place, rather than simply redistributing welfare as a post hoc remedy to entrenched systemic inequality.

Such a model of neorepublican social democracy for the twenty-first century will not only be necessary to promote freedom as non-domination, neutralising the opportunities for economically and socially powerful agents to wield discretionary power over others, it will also help to promote increased resilience to crises; proactively seeking to mitigate and avert such threats to common wellbeing. The pandemic, the cost of living crisis, the climate emergency: each of these crises risks creating opportunities for the advantaged, the wealthy, and the powerful to dominate, exploit, and manipulate the poor, the precarious, and the vulnerable. Neorepublicans are therefore predisposed to keep a weather eye on the lookout for potential threats, and to endorse utilising the full potential of the democratic state to pre-emptively limit the risks of calamitous social, economic, or environmental crisis (e.g. by maintaining good levels of public health, providing state support to a faltering economy, and by coordinating a just transition away from carbon-intensive ways of life), and respond dynamically and forcefully when necessary.

In other words, neorepublican social democracy offers a complete counterpoint to the neoliberal approach—a truly *antineoliberal* alternative—that promotes action over inaction, citizenship over consumerism, and equality over inequality in pursuit of shared freedom within a free state.

Conclusion

This book has offered a revelatory, explanatory, and now instructive exploration of the UK's deleterious encounter with the COVID-19 pandemic. This case study has emphasised the extent to which this can be understood as a distinctly *political* pandemic and not a solely natural disaster, the scale and severity of which was somehow beyond human control. Constrained by the logics and legacies of hegemonic neoliberal ideology, the British state has exposed its citizens to extraordinary harms, and proven insufficiently resilient to crisis. Any public inquiry must now consider these contingent political and philosophical factors as we collectively attempt to learn the lessons of our failure to limit the impacts of COVID-19. The pandemic was not just an accident of poor decision-making in the moment, it was a predictable consequence of the inertia, impotence, and inequality nurtured by the state, both during the pandemic itself and over the preceding forty years of neoliberal policymaking.

In making this case, we have attempted to exhibit the critical potential of cross-disciplinary collaboration, as well as applied political theory as a methodology. By isolating and interrogating the political theoretical ideas and commitments that have underpinned neoliberal policymaking in the UK—in particular a conception of freedom as non-interference—we have been able to provide a systematic challenge to these ideas from both a political and practical angle. Not only are the neoliberal instincts at the heart of current UK policymaking politically contingent (i.e. neither natural, nor inevitable), they are also both unjust and unnecessary. Without this level of political theoretical interrogation, it would be impossible to fully understand the underlying, long-term drivers of political decision-making during the pandemic. From this vantage point, we can more clearly see that any failure of the UK to protect lives and livelihoods from COVID-19 is the consequence not just of particular, incompetent policymakers and the various mistakes they may have made during the pandemic, but of a constrained choice architecture cultivated over decades thanks to a hegemonic commitment to orthodox neoliberal thought.

Further work now is required to flesh out how neoliberalism can be effectively dismantled and discarded as the UK, and the world, seeks to recover and rebuild resilience in the wake of the pandemic. But this is not a time for complacency, it is a time for action and a time for change. Only by challenging neoliberal hegemony can we truly build back better.

References

Barry, J. (2021). Green republicanism and a 'Just Transition' from the tyranny of economic growth. *Critical Review of International Social and Political Philosophy, 24*(5), 725–742.

Cumbers, A. (2020). *The case for economic democracy*. Polity Press Bristol.

Dean, J. (2009). Democracy and other neoliberal fantasies. In *Democracy and other neoliberal fantasies*. Duke University Press.

Hansard, H. C. (2022, April 27). Deb (vol. 712, col. 755).

Harvey. (2005). *A brief history of neoliberalism*. Oxford University Press.

HM Government. (2022). Covid-19 response: Living with Covid-19. https://assets.publishing.service.gov.uk/government/uploads/system/uploads/attachment_data/file/1056229/COVID-19_Response_-_Living_with_COVID-19.pdf. Accessed 12 May 2022.

HM Treasury. (2022). Government support for the cost of living: Factsheet. https://www.gov.uk/government/publications/government-support-for-the-cost-of-living-factsheet/government-support-for-the-cost-of-living-fac tsheet. Accessed 12 May 2022.

Klein, N. (2020). *On fire: The (burning) case for a green new deal*. Simon & Schuster.

Institute for Government. (2022). Cost of living crisis. https://www.institutefor government.org.uk/explainers/cost-living-crisis. Accessed 12 May 2022.

Intergovernmental Panel on Climate Change [IPCC]. (2022). Climate Change 2022 mitigation of Climate Change: Summary for policymakers. https://report.ipcc.ch/ar6wg3/pdf/IPCC_AR6_WGIII_Summar yForPolicymakers.pdf. Accessed 12 May 2022.

Lefkowitz, D. (2014). Strains of commitment. In J. Mandle & D. A. Reidy (Eds.), *The Cambridge Rawls Lexicon* (pp. 813–816). Cambridge University Press.

Leipold, B., Nabulsi, K., & White, S. (2020). *Radical republicanism: Recovering the tradition's popular heritage*. Oxford University Press.

Mouffe, C. (2000). *The democratic paradox*. Verso.

Mouffe, C. (2005). *On the political*. Routledge.

Mouffe, C. (2013). *Agonistics*. Verso.

Painter, A. (2020). Coronavirus: Respond at scale, build bridges to the future. https://www.thersa.org/blog/2020/03/coronavirus-respond-at-scale-build-bridges-to-the-future. Accessed 12 May 2022.

Pettit, P. (1997). *Republicanism: A theory of freedom and government*. Oxford University Press.

Pettit, P. (2002). Keeping republican freedom simple: On a difference with Quentin Skinner. *Political Theory, 30*(3), 339–356.

Pettit, P. (2010). Civic republican theory. In J. L. Martí & P. Pettit (Eds.), *A political philosophy in public life: Civic republicanism in Zapatero's Spain*. Princeton University Press.

Ranciere, J. (1995). *On the shores of politics*. Verso.

Ranciere, J. (1999). *Disagreement: Politics and philosophy*. University of Minnesota Press.

Ranciere, J. (2006). *Hatred of democracy*. Verso.

Rawls, J. (2001). *Justice as fairness: A restatement*. Harvard University Press.

Raworth, K. (2017). *Doughnut economics: Seven ways to think like a 21st-century economist*. Chelsea Green Publishing.

Resolution Foundation. (2022). Inflation nation: Putting spring statement 2022 in context. https://www.resolutionfoundation.org/publications/inflation-nat ion/. Accessed 12 May 2022.

Roy, A. (2020). The pandemic is a portal. https://www.ft.com/content/10d 8f5e8-74eb-11ea-95fe-fcd274e920ca. Accessed 12 May 2022.

Skinner, Q. (2012). *Liberty before liberalism*. Cambridge University Press.

Swyngedouw, E. (2009). The antinomies of the postpolitical city: In search of a democratic politics of environmental production. *International Journal of Urban and Regional Research, 33*(3), 601e620.

Žižek, S. (1999). *The Ticklish subject: The absent centre of political ontology*. Verso.

Appendix

Table A1 Guide to Western (leaning) geographical units/territorial blocs referred to in Chapter 3

Theme	Geographical units of analysis and associated data sets
Global base data	**UN Member States n = 193 Total population = 7.85 billion (mid 2021) The United Kingdom (UK) Total population 0.068 billion** The United Nations member states are the 193 sovereign states that are members of the United Nations (UN) and have equal representation in the UN General Assembly

(continued)

Table A1 (continued)

Theme	Geographical units of analysis and associated data sets
	Afghanistan, Albania, Algeria, Andorra, Angola, Antigua and Barbuda, Argentina, Armenia, Australia, Austria, Azerbaijan, Bahrain, Bangladesh, Barbados, Belarus, Belgium, Belize, Benin, Bhutan, Bolivia, Bosnia and Herzegovina, Botswana, Brazil, Brunei, Bulgaria, Burkina Faso, Burundi, Cambodia, Cameroon, Canada, Cape Verde, Central African Republic, Chad, Chile, China, Colombia, Comoros, Costa Rica, Croatia, Cuba, Cyprus, Czech Republic (Czechia), Democratic Republic of the Congo, Denmark, Djibouti, Dominica, Dominican Republic, East Timor, Ecuador, Egypt, El Salvador, Equatorial Guinea, Eritrea, Estonia, Eswatini, Ethiopia, Fiji, Finland, France, Gabon, Georgia, Germany, Ghana, Greece, Grenada, Guatemala, Guinea, Guinea-Bissau, Guyana, Haiti, Honduras, Hungary, Iceland, India, Indonesia, Iran, Iraq, Ireland, Israel, Italy, Ivory Coast, Jamaica, Japan, Jordan, Kazakhstan, Kenya, Kiribati, Kuwait, Kyrgyzstan, Laos, Latvia, Lebanon, Lesotho, Liberia, Libya, Liechtenstein, Lithuania, Luxembourg, Madagascar, Malawi, Malaysia, Maldives, Mali, Malta, Marshall Islands, Mauritania, Mauritius, Mexico, Moldova, Monaco, Mongolia, Montenegro, Morocco, Mozambique, Myanmar, Namibia, Nauru, Nepal, Netherlands, New Zealand, Nicaragua, Niger, Nigeria, North Korea, North Macedonia, Norway, Oman, Pakistan, Palau, Panama, Papua New Guinea, Paraguay, Peru, Philippines, Poland, Portugal, Qatar, Republic of the Congo, Romania, Russia, Rwanda, Saint Kitts and Nevis, Saint Lucia, Saint Vincent and the Grenadines, Samoa, San Marino, São Tomé and Príncipe, Saudi Arabia, Senegal, Serbia, Seychelles, Sierra Leone, Singapore, Slovakia, Slovenia, Solomon Islands, Somalia, South Africa, South Korea, South Sudan, Spain, Sri Lanka, Sudan, Suriname, Sweden, Switzerland, Syria, Tajikistan, Tanzania, Thailand, The Bahamas, the Federated States of Micronesia, The Gambia, Togo, Tonga, Trinidad and Tobago, Tunisia, Turkey, Turkmenistan, Tuvalu, Uganda, Ukraine, United Arab Emirates, United Kingdom, United States, Uruguay, Uzbekistan, Vanuatu, Venezuela, Vietnam, Yemen, Zambia, Zimbabwe
Health	**WHO European Region countries $n = 53$ Total population 0.89 billion** The WHO Regional Office for Europe (WHO/Europe) is one of WHO's six regional offices around the world. It serves the WHO European Region, which comprises 53 countries, covering a geographical region from the Atlantic to the Pacific oceans

(continued)

Table A1   (continued)

Theme	Geographical units of analysis and associated data sets
	Albania Andorra Armenia Austria Azerbaijan Belarus Belgium Bosnia and Herzegovina Bulgaria Croatia Cyprus Czechia Denmark Estonia Finland France Georgia Germany Greece Hungary Iceland Ireland Israel Italy Kazakhstan Kyrgyzstan Latvia Lithuania Luxembourg Malta Monaco Montenegro Netherlands North Poland Portugal Republic of Moldova Romania Russian Federation San Marino Serbia Slovakia Slovenia Spain Sweden Switzerland Tajikistan Turkey Turkmenistan Ukraine United Kingdom of Great Britain and Northern Ireland Uzbekistan
Economy, Development, Income	**World Bank High Income countries** n **= 80 Total population = 1.27 billion (2022)** The World Bank assigns the world's economies to four income groups—low, lower-middle, upper-middle, and high-income countries. The classifications are updated each year on July 1 and are based on GNI per capita in current USD (using the Atlas method exchange rates) of the previous year (i.e. 2021 in this case). High income countries are countries with GNI per capita > US$12,695 Andorra Antigua and Barbuda Aruba Australia Austria Bahamas, The Bahrain Barbados Belgium Bermuda British Virgin Islands Brunei Darussalam Canada Cayman Islands Channel Islands Chile Croatia Curaçao Cyprus Czech Republic Denmark Estonia Faroe Islands Finland France French Polynesia Germany Gibraltar Greece Greenland Guam Hong Kong SAR, China Hungary Iceland Ireland Isle of Man Israel Italy Japan Korea, Rep. Kuwait Latvia Liechtenstein Lithuania Luxembourg Macao SAR, China Malta Monaco Nauru Netherlands New Caledonia New Zealand Northern Mariana Islands Norway Oman Palau Poland Portugal Puerto Rico Qatar San Marino Saudi Arabia Seychelles Singapore Sint Maarten (Dutch part) Slovak Republic Slovenia Spain St. Kitts and Nevis St. Martin (French part) Sweden Switzerland Taiwan, China Trinidad and Tobago Turks and Caicos Islands United Arab Emirates United Kingdom United States Uruguay Virgin Islands (U.S.) **United Nations Human Development Index** n **= 30 (top ranked countries) Total population = 0.89 billion** The Human Development Index (HDI) is a measure of countries level of human development based upon life expectancy, education (mean years of schooling completed and expected years of schooling upon entering the education system), and per capita income indicators Australia Austria Belgium Canada Cyprus Czechia Denmark Estonia Finland France Germany Hong Kong Iceland Ireland Israel Italy Japan Liechtenstein Luxembourg Malta Netherlands New Zealand Norway Singapore Slovenia South Korea Spain Sweden Switzerland United Kingdom United States **International Monetary Fund (IMF) Advanced Economies** n **= 40 Total population 1.1 billion**

(continued)

Table A1   (continued)

Theme	Geographical units of analysis and associated data sets
	The IMF use the label advanced economy to describe the most developed countries in the world—referring therein to countries with high levels of per capita income, a varied export base, and a financial sector that's integrated into the global financial system
	Andorra Australia Austria Belgium Canada Cyprus Czech Republic Denmark Estonia Finland France Germany Greece Hong Kong SAR Iceland Ireland Israel Italy Japan S Korea Latvia Lithuania Luxembourg Macao SAR Malta Netherlands New Zealand Norway Portugal Puerto Rico San Marino Singapore Slovak Republic Slovenia Spain Sweden Switzerland Taiwan United Kingdom United States
	The Organisation for Economic Co-operation and Development (OECD) Advanced Liberal Market Democracies n = 38 Total population 1.36 billion
	The OECD comprises 38 countries committed to improving public policy within the framework of liberal market democracy
	Australia Austria Belgium Canada Chile Colombia Costa Rica Czech Republic Denmark Estonia Finland France Germany Greece Hungary Iceland Ireland Israel Italy Japan South Korea Latvia Lithuania Luxembourg Mexico Netherlands New Zealand Norway Poland Portugal Slovak Republic Slovenia Spain Sweden Switzerland Turkey United Kingdom United States
Democracy, Liberalism, Freedom	**V-Dem Institute Liberal Democracy Index (LDI) and Regimes of Democracy** n = 34 Total population 1.3 billion
	The V-Dem Liberal Democracy Index (LDI) captures both liberal and electoral aspects of democracy based on an exhaustive set of indicators. Countries defined as supporting a Liberal Democracy Regime of Democracy are assumed to be most free and democratic
	Australia Barbados Belgium Bhutan Botswana Canada Chile Costa Rica Cyprus Denmark Estonia Finland France Germany Greece Iceland Ireland Israel Italy Japan Latvia Luxembourg Netherlands New Zealand Norway Portugal Seychelles South Korea Spain Sweden Switzerland Taiwan United Kingdom United States Uruguay
	Cato Institute/Fraser Institute Human Freedom Index 2021 n = 30 Total population 0.95 billion
	Published by the US Cato Institute and Canadian Fraser Institute uses 82 indicators of personal and economic freedom to measure the extent to which countries can be defined as libertarian. The top 30 (free-ist) countries are examined in this book
	Australia Austria Belgium Canada Chile Cyprus Czechia Denmark Estonia Finland Germany Hong Kong Iceland Ireland Italy Japan Latvia Lithuania Luxembourg Malta Netherlands New Zealand Norway Portugal Spain Sweden Switzerland Taiwan United Kingdom United States
	DHL Global Connectivity Index n = 30 Total population 1.32 billion

(continued)

Table A1   (continued)

Theme	*Geographical units of analysis and associated data sets*
	The DHL Global Connectedness Index measures globalization based on international trade, capital, information, and people flows. It is unique in that it tracks both the size of countries' international flows relative to their domestic activity ("depth") and their geographic reach around the world ("breadth")
	Austria Belgium Cyprus Czechia Denmark Estonia Finland France Germany Hong Kong Hungary Iceland Ireland Israel Italy Japan Luxembourg Malaysia Malta Netherlands Singapore Slovenia South Korea Spain Sweden Switzerland Taiwan Thailand United Kingdom United States
	Economist Democracy Index n = 30 (top 30 most democratic) Total population 0.98 billion
	The Democracy Index is based on 60 indicators, grouped into five categories: electoral process and pluralism, civil liberties, functioning of government, political participation and political culture
	Australia Austria Botswana Canada Chile Costa Rica Czechia Denmark Estonia Finland France Germany Iceland Ireland Israel Japan Luxembourg Mauritius Netherlands New Zealand Norway Portugal South Korea Spain Sweden Switzerland Taiwan United Kingdom United States Uruguay
Power, Influence, Leadership	**North Atlantic Treaty Organisation (NATO) n = 30 Total population 0.94 billion**
	NATO is an intergovernmental military alliance between 30 'western alliance' member states—28 European and 2 North American
	Albania Belgium Bulgaria Canada Croatia Czechia Denmark Estonia France Germany Greece Hungary Ireland Italy Latvia Lithuania Luxembourg Montenegro Netherlands North Macedonia Norway Poland Portugal Romania Slovakia Slovenia Spain Turkey United Kingdom United States
	European Union EU27 n = 27 Total population
	European Union EU27 n = 27 Total population 0.45 billion
	The European Union (EU) is a political and economic union of 27 member states
	Austria Belgium Bulgaria Croatia Cyprus Czechia Denmark Estonia Finland France Germany Greece Hungary Ireland Italy Latvia Lithuania Luxembourg Malta Netherlands Poland Portugal Romania Slovakia Slovenia Spain Sweden
	G20 World's Largest Advanced And Emerging Economies n = 19 + EU Total population 4.7 billion

(continued)

Table A1   (continued)

Theme	Geographical units of analysis and associated data sets
	The G20 or Group of Twenty is an intergovernmental forum comprising 19 countries and the European Union (EU). It works to address major issues related to the global economy Argentina Australia Brazil Canada China France Germany India Indonesia Italy Japan Republic of Korea Mexico Russia Saudi Arabia South Africa Turkey United Kingdom United States European Union **G7 Major Advanced Economies** n **= 7 Total Population 700 million + EU** The G7 or Group of 7 is an intergovernmental forum comprising 7 leading western nations. It works to address major issues related to the global economy Canada France Germany Italy Japan United Kingdom United States **The Paris Club** n **= 22 Total population 1.32 billion** The Paris Club comprises major creditor countries whose role is to find co-ordinated and sustainable solutions to the payment difficulties experienced by debtor countries Australia Austria Belgium Brazil Canada Denmark Finland France Germany Ireland Israel Italy Japan Norway Russia South Korea Spain Sweden Switzerland United Kingdom United States **Portland 30 Soft Power Index** n **= 30 Total population 4.3 billion** The Portland 30 index measures the degree of soft power countries are able to mobilise to leverage the international system. It combines both objective data across six categories (Government, Culture, Education, Global Engagement, Enterprise, and Digital) and international polling. It identifies the top 30 'nation brands', Australia Austria Belgium Brazil Canada China Czechia Denmark Finland France Germany Greece Hungary India Ireland Italy Japan Netherlands New Zealand Norway Poland Portugal Russia Singapore South Korea Sweden Switzerland Turkey United Kingdom United States
Imperialism, History, Culture	**Large Anglophone countries** n **= 7 Total population 0.55 billion** Seven large English speak countries with historical ties to the UK United Kingdom United States Canada, Australia, Ireland New Zealand South Africa

Table A2a–e Placing the advanced capitalist world in global context

(a) *% share of world's confirmed COVID-19 deaths by territorial bloc Jan 2020–June 2022*

	Health	Economy, Development, Income				Democracy, Liberalism, Freedom				Power, Influence, Leadership						Imperialism, History, Culture	
	WHO European Region (%)	World Bank High Income Region (%)	UN Very High HDI (%)	IMF Advanced Economies (%)	OECD (%)	VDEm Liberal Democracies (%)	Cato/Fraser Human Freedom Index (%)	DHL Global Connectivity Index (%)	Economist Full Democracies (%)	NATO (%)	EU27 (%)	G20 (%)	G7 (%)	Paris Club (%)	Portland 30 (%)	Anglophone (%)	UK (%)
% of Global Population	9.50	15.50	11.40	14.20	18.00	13.6	12.1	9.7	12.8	12.2	9.8	64.0	10.0	17.0	55.0	7.0	0.8
% share of world's confirmed COVID-19 deaths																	
Jan 1 2020 to June 30 2020	36.6	59.3	60.0	58.8	64.6	58.1	52.7	31.8	50.1	57.0	24.6	96.2	40.1	69.8	70.4	34.7	7.5
Jan 1 2020 to Dec 31 2020	32.5	44.4	39.8	43.7	52.0	40.2	37.3	20.8	36.0	43.6	19.7	87.3	28.9	52.3	62.0	26.1	3.9
Jan 1 2021 to Dec 31 2021	47.3	38.0	25.6	30.6	36.9	26.5	24.8	14.1	24.8	32.5	15.2	79.4	20.3	43.6	57.6	18.4	2.1
Jan 1 2022 to June 30 2022	35.9	56.1	47.3	53.1	57.0	49.9	31.1	26.1	45.6	49.2	21.9	89.7	34.7	58.8	57.0	30.9	3.5
Jan 1 2020 to June 30 2022	32.0	38.5	32.7	37.5	44.0	33.7	31.4	17.6	30.1	38.0	17.4	83.1	24.7	48.1	68.7	22.3	2.8

(continued)

Table A2a–e (continued)

(b) % share of world's excess deaths by territorial bloc Jan 2020–Jun 2022

	Health	Economy, Development, Income				Democracy, Liberalism, Freedom				Power, Influence, Leadership						Imperialism, History, Culture	
	WHO European Region (%)	World Bank High Income Region (%)	UN Very High HDI (%)	IMF Advanced Economies (%)	OECD (%)	VDEm Liberal Democracies (%)	Cato/Fraser Human Freedom Index (%)	DHL Global Connectivity Index (%)	Economist Full Democracies (%)	NATO (%)	EU27 (%)	G20 (%)	G7 (%)	Paris Club (%)	Portland 30 (%)	Anglophone (%)	UK (%)
% of Global Population	9.50	15.50	11.40	14.20	18.00	13.60	12.10	9.70	12.80	12.20	9.80	64.00	10.00	17.00	55.00	7.00	0.80
% share of world's excess deaths																	
Jan 1 2020 to June 30 2020	24.1	31.6	29.0	29.7	39.6	29.6	28.2	27.8	24.7	32.5	17.4	66.3	18.9	39.6	55.5	18.2	4.8
Jan 1 2020 to Dec 31 2020	22.7	20.1	17.2	19.5	28.0	17.1	16.6	17.0	15.1	7.2	10.7	68.2	12.2	27.1	56.2	11.8	1.5
Jan 1 2021 to Dec 31 2021	15.8	10.3	7.7	9.4	14.6	8.0	10.5	8.5	7.5	11.8	4.7	65.4	6.0	17.2	55.7	6.4	0.4
Jan 1 2022 to June 30 2022	11.7	12.5	10.2	11.2	14.9	11.1	9.5	11.2	10.2	10.2	3.4	62.0	7.5	17.8	53.4	6.0	0.2
Jan 1 2020 to June 30 2022	17.1	13.5	10.7	12.5	18.3	11.1	10.5	11.3	10.0	14.4	6.1	65.6	8.0	20.0	55.5	7.8	0.7

(c) Ratio (in %) of actual % share of world's confirmed COVID-19 deaths relative to % share of COVID-19 deaths which would have occurred had COVID-19 spread evenly varying only by population size by territorial bloc Jan 2020–June 2022

	Health	Economy, Development, Income				Democracy, Liberalism, Freedom				Power, Influence, Leadership						Imperialism, History, Culture	
	WHO European Region (%)	World Bank High Income Region (%)	UN Very High HDI (%)	IMF Advanced Economies (%)	OECD (%)	VDEm Liberal Democracies (%)	Cato/Fraser Human Freedom Index (%)	DHL Global Connectivity Index (%)	Economist Full Democracies (%)	NATO (%)	EU27 (%)	G20 (%)	G7 (%)	Paris Club (%)	Portland 30 (%)	Anglophone (%)	UK (%)
% of Global Population	9.5	15.5	11.4	14.2	18.0	13.6	12.1	9.7	12.8	12.2	9.8	64.0	10.0	17.0	55.0	7.0	0.8
Ratio (in %) of actual % share of world's confirmed COVID-19 deaths relative to % share of COVID-19 deaths which would have occurred had COVID-19 spread evenly varying only by population size																	
Jan 1 2020 to June 30 2020	385.3	382.6	526.3	414.1	358.9	427.2	435.5	327.8	391.4	467.2	251.0	150.3	401.0	410.6	128.0	495.7	937.5
Jan 1 2020 to Dec 31 2020	342.1	286.5	349.1	307.7	288.9	295.6	308.3	214.4	281.3	357.4	201.0	136.4	289.0	307.6	112.7	372.9	487.5
Jan 1 2021 to Dec 31 2021	497.9	245.2	224.6	215.5	205.0	194.9	205.0	145.4	193.8	266.4	155.1	124.1	203.0	256.5	104.7	262.9	262.5
Jan 1 2022 to June 30 2022	377.9	361.9	414.9	373.9	316.7	366.9	257.0	269.1	356.3	403.3	223.5	140.2	347.0	345.9	103.6	441.4	437.5
Jan 1 2020 to June 30 2022	336.8	248.4	286.8	264.1	244.4	247.8	259.5	181.4	235.2	311.5	177.6	129.8	247.0	282.9	124.9	318.6	350.0

(continued)

Table A2a–e (continued)

(d) Ratio (in %) of actual % share of world's excess deaths relative to % share of excess deaths which would have occurred had COVID-19 spread evenly varying only by population size by territorial bloc Jan 2020–June 2022

	Health	Economy, Development, Income				Democracy, Liberalism, Freedom				Power, Influence, Leadership						Imperialism, History, Culture	
	WHO European Region (%)	World Bank Income Region (%)	UN Very High HDI (%)	IMF Advanced Economies (%)	OECD (%)	VDem Liberal Democracies (%)	Cato/ Fraser Human Freedom Index (%)	DHL Global Connectivity Index (%)	Economist Full Democracies (%)	NATO (%)	EU (%)	G20 (%)	G7 (%)	Paris Club (%)	Portland 30 (%)	Anglophone (%)	UK (%)
% of Global Population	9.5	15.5	11.4	14.2	18.0	13.6	12.1	9.7	12.8	12.2	9.8	64.0	10.0	17.0	55.0	7.0	0.8
Jan 1 2020 to June 30 2020	253.7	203.9	254.4	209.2	220.0	217.6	233.1	286.6	193.0	266.4	177.6	103.6	189.0	232.9	100.9	260.0	600.0
Jan 1 2020 to Dec 31 2020	238.9	129.7	150.9	137.3	155.6	125.7	137.2	175.3	118.0	59.0	109.2	106.6	122.0	159.4	102.2	168.6	187.5
Jan 1 2021 to Dec 31 2021	166.3	66.5	67.5	66.2	81.1	58.8	86.8	87.6	58.6	96.7	48.0	102.2	60.0	101.2	101.3	91.4	50.0
Jan 1 2022 to June 30 2022	123.2	80.6	89.5	78.9	82.8	59.0	78.5	115.5	79.7	83.6	34.7	96.9	75.0	104.7	97.1	85.7	25.0
Jan 1 2020 to June 30 2022	180.0	87.1	93.9	88.0	101.7	81.6	86.8	116.5	78.1	118.0	62.2	102.5	80.0	117.6	100.9	111.4	87.5

Ratio (in %) of actual % share of world's deaths relative to %excess share of excess deaths which would have occurred had COVID-19 spread evenly varying only by population size

(e) Ratio of % share of confirmed COVID-19 deaths relative to % share of world's excess deaths by territorial bloc Jan 2020–June 2022

	Health Economy, Development, Income					Democracy, Liberalism, Freedom				Power, Influence, Leadership						Imperialism, History, Culture	
	WHO European Region (%)	World Bank Income Region (%)	UN Very High HDI (%)	IMF Advanced Economies (%)	OECD (%)	VDEm Liberal Democracies (%)	Cato/Fraser Human Freedom Index (%)	DHL Global Connectivity Index (%)	Economist Full Democracies (%)	NATO (%)	EU (%)	G20 (%)	G7 (%)	Paris Club (%)	Portland 30 (%)	Anglophone (%)	UK (%)
% of Global Population	9.50	15.50	11.40	14.20	18.00	13.60	12.10	9.70	12.80	12.20	9.80	64.00	10.00	17.00	55.00	7.00	0.80
Ratio of % share of world's confirmed COVID-19 deaths relative to % share of world's excess deaths																	
Jan 1 2020 to June 30 2020	1.5	1.9	2.1	2.0	1.6	2.0	1.9	1.1	2.0	1.8	1.4	1.5	2.1	1.8	1.3	1.9	1.6
Jan 1 2020 to Dec 31 2020	1.4	2.2	2.3	2.2	1.9	2.4	2.2	1.2	2.4	6.1	1.8	1.3	2.4	1.9	1.1	2.2	2.6
Jan 1 2021 to Dec 31 2021	3.0	3.7	3.3	3.3	2.5	3.3	2.4	1.7	3.3	2.8	3.2	1.2	3.4	2.5	1.0	2.9	5.3
Jan 1 2022 to June 30 2022	3.1	4.5	4.6	4.7	3.8	4.5	3.3	2.3	4.5	4.8	6.4	1.4	4.6	3.3	1.1	5.2	17.5
Jan 1 2020 to June 30 2022	1.9	2.9	3.1	3.0	2.4	3.0	3.0	1.6	3.0	2.6	2.9	1.3	3.1	2.4	1.2	2.9	4.0

Source John Hopkins University Center for Systems Science and Engineering (CSSE) COVID-19 Data Repository and The Economist excess deaths tracker - https://www.economist.com/graphic-detail/coronavirus-excess-deaths-tracker

Table A3a–e Placing the UK in the context of a range highly developed liberal market democratic territorial blocs

(a) The UKs % share of confirmed COVID-19 deaths by territorial bloc Jan 2020–June 2022

	Health		Economy, Development, Income				Democracy, Liberalism, Freedom				Power, Influence, Leadership						Imperialism, History, Culture
	Global (%)	WHO European Region (%)	World Bank High Income Region (%)	UN Very High HDI (%)	IMF Advanced Economies (%)	OECD (%)	VDEm Liberal Democracies (%)	Cato/Fraser Human Freedom Index (%)	DHL Global Connectivity Index (%)	Economist Full Democracies (%)	NATO (%)	EU27 (%)	G20 (%)	G7 (%)	Paris Club (%)	Portland 30 (%)	Anglophone (%)
UKs % share of population	0.8	10.9	5.0	7.7	6.2	5.1	6.3	7.2	11.1	6.8	7.1	13.2	1.5	9.9	5.1	1.6	12.8
UKs % share of confirmed COVID-19 Deaths by territorial bloc																	
Jan 1 2020 to June 30 2020	7.5	20.4	12.6	13.1	12.7	11.6	12.9	14.2	23.5	14.9	13.1	30.4	7.8	16.1	10.7	10.6	21.6
Jan 1 2020 to Dec 31 2020	3.9	12.1	8.9	9.9	8.8	7.5	9.8	10.5	18.9	11.0	9.0	19.8	4.5	12.0	7.5	6.4	15.7
Jan 1 2021 to Dec 31 2021	2.1	4.5	6.8	8.3	7.0	5.8	8.1	8.6	15.1	10.9	6.6	14.1	2.7	9.7	4.9	3.7	11.6
Jan 1 2022 to June 30 2022	3.5	9.8	6.3	7.5	6.7	6.2	7.0	7.8	13.5	8.6	7.2	16.1	3.9	9.5	6.0	5.1	11.5
Jan 1 2020 to June 30 2022	2.8	8.9	6.5	8.7	7.5	6.5	8.4	9.0	16.0	9.2	7.5	16.3	3.4	10.4	5.9	4.7	12.7

(b) The UK's % share of excess deaths by territorial bloc Jan 2020–Jun 2022

	Global (%)	Health	Economy, Development, Income				Democracy, Liberalism, Freedom				Power, Influence, Leadership						Imperialism, History, Culture
		WHO European Region (%)	World Bank High Income Region (%)	UN Very High HDI (%)	IMF Advanced Economics (%)	OECD (%)	VDEm Liberal Democracies (%)	Cato/Fraser Human Freedom Index (%)	DHL Global Connectivity Index (%)	Economist Full Democracies (%)	NATO (%)	EU27 (%)	G20 (%)	G7 (%)	Paris Club (%)	Portland 30 (%)	Anglophone (%)
UK % of Population	0.8	10.9	5.5	7.7	6.2	5.1	6.3	7.2	11.1	6.8	7.1	13.2	1.5	9.9	5.1	1.6	12.8
UK's % share of excess deaths by territorial bloc																	
Jan 1 2020 to June 30 2020	4.8	20.7	15.8	17.1	16.8	12.6	16.9	17.6	17.9	20.2	15.4	28.5	7.5	26.4	12.6	5.0	27.3
Jan 1 2020 to Dec 31 2020	1.5	7.0	7.7	9.3	8.2	5.7	9.3	9.6	9.4	10.5	7.2	15.0	2.3	13.0	5.9	1.6	13.5
Jan 1 2021 to Dec 31 2021	0.4	3.0	4.6	6.2	5.0	3.2	5.9	6.2	5.6	6.4	4.0	10.2	0.7	7.9	2.8	0.5	7.5
Jan 1 2022 to June 30 2022	0.2	1.4	1.3	1.6	1.4	1.1	1.5	1.7	1.4	1.6	1.6	4.9	0.3	2.2	1.1	0.3	2.7
Jan 1 2020 to June 30 2022	0.7	4.3	5.4	6.8	5.9	4.0	6.6	7.0	6.5	7.3	5.1	12.0	1.1	9.2	3.7	0.7	9.3

(continued)

Table A3a–e (continued)

(c) Ratio (in %) of UKs % share of confirmed COVID-19 deaths relative to the % share of COVID-19 deaths UK would have had had COVID-19 spread evenly over the earth's surface varying only by population size, by territorial bloc Jan 2020–June 2022

	Health		Economy, Development, Income				Democracy, Liberalism, Freedom				Power, Influence, Leadership						Imperialism, History, Culture
	Global (%)	WHO European Region (%)	World Bank High Income Region (%)	UN Very High HDI (%)	IMF Advanced Economies (%)	OECD (%)	VDem Liberal Democracies (%)	Cato/Fraser Human Freedom Index (%)	DHL Global Connectivity Index (%)	Economist Full Democracies (%)	NATO (%)	EU27 (%)	G20 (%)	G7 (%)	Paris Club (%)	Portland 30 (%)	Anglophone (%)
UK % of Population	0.8	10.9	5.0	7.7	6.2	5.1	6.3	7.2	11.1	6.8	7.1	13.2	1.5	9.9	5.1	1.6	12.8
Ratio (in %)—UKs % share of confirmed COVID-19 deaths relative to % share of confirmed COVID-19 deaths UK would have had had COVID-19 spread evenly over the earth's surface varying only by population size, by territorial bloc																	
Jan 1 2020 to June 30 2020	937.5	187.2	252.0	170.1	204.8	227.5	204.8	197.2	211.7	219.1	184.5	230.3	520.0	162.6	209.8	662.5	168.8
Jan 1 2020 to Dec 31 2020	487.5	111.0	178.0	128.6	141.9	147.1	155.6	145.8	170.3	161.8	126.8	150.0	300.0	121.2	147.1	400.0	122.7
Jan 1 2021 to Dec 31 2021	262.5	41.3	136.0	107.8	112.9	113.7	128.6	119.4	136.0	160.3	93.0	106.8	60.0	98.0	96.1	231.3	90.6
Jan 1 2022 to June 30 2022	437.5	89.9	126.0	97.4	108.1	121.6	111.1	108.3	121.6	126.5	101.4	122.0	#REF!	96.0	117.6	318.8	89.8
Jan 1 2020 to June 30 2022	350.0	81.7	130.0	113.0	121.0	127.5	133.3	125.0	144.1	135.3	105.6	123.5	226.7	105.1	115.7	293.8	99.2

(d) Ratio (in %) of UKs % share of excess deaths relative to the % share of excess deaths UK would have had COVID-19 spread evenly over the earth's surface varying only by population size, by territorial bloc Jan 2020–June 2022

		Health	Economy, Development, Income					Democracy, Liberalism, Freedom				Power, Influence, Leadership						Imperialism, History, Culture
	Global (%)	WHO European Region (%)	World Bank High Income Region (%)	UN Very High HDI (%)	IMF Advanced Economies (%)	OECD (%)	VDEm Liberal Democracies (%)	Cato/Fraser Human Freedom Index (%)	DHL Global Connectivity Index (%)	Economist Full Democracies (%)	NATO (%)	EU27 (%)	G20 (%)	G7 (%)	Paris Club (%)	Portland 30 (%)	Anglophone (%)
UK % of Population	0.8	10.9	5.5	7.7	6.2	5.1	6.3	7.2	11.1	6.8	7.1	13.2	1.5	9.9	5.1	1.6	12.8
Ratio (in %)—UKs % share of excess deaths relative to % share of excess deaths UK would have had COVID-19 spread evenly over the earth's surface varying only by population size, by territorial bloc																	
Jan 1 2020 to June 30 2020	600.0	189.9	287.3	222.1	271.0	247.1	268.3	244.4	161.3	297.1	216.9	215.9	500.0	266.7	247.1	312.5	213.3
Jan 1 2020 to Dec 31 2020	187.5	64.2	140.0	120.8	132.3	111.8	147.6	133.3	84.7	154.4	101.4	113.6	153.3	131.3	115.7	100.0	105.5
Jan 1 2021 to Dec 31 2021	50.0	27.5	83.6	80.5	80.6	62.7	93.7	86.1	50.5	94.1	56.3	77.3	46.7	79.8	54.9	31.3	58.6
Jan 1 2022 to June 30 2022	25.0	12.8	23.6	20.8	22.6	21.6	23.8	23.6	12.6	23.5	22.5	37.1	20.0	22.2	21.6	18.8	21.1
Jan 1 2020 to June 30 2022	87.5	39.4	98.2	88.3	95.2	78.4	104.8	97.2	58.6	107.4	71.8	90.9	73.3	92.9	72.5	43.8	72.7

(continued)

Table A3a–e (continued)

(e) Ratio of UKs % share of confirmed COVID-19 deaths relative to UKs % share of world's excess deaths, by territorial bloc Jan 2020 to June 2022

UKs % share of confirmed COVID-19 deaths relative to % share of excess deaths, by territorial bloc

UKs % share of confirmed COVID-19 deaths relative to % share of confirmed COVID-19 deaths, by territorial bloc

	Global (%)	Health	Economy, Development, Income					Democracy, Liberalism, Freedom				Power, Influence, Leadership						Imperialism, History, Culture
		WHO European Region (%)	World Bank High Income Region (%)	UN Very High HDI (%)	IMF Advanced Economies (%)	OECD (%)	VDEm Liberal Democracies (%)	Cato/Fraser Human Freedom Index (%)	DHL Global Connectivity Index (%)	Economist Full Democracies (%)	NATO (%)	EU27 (%)	G20 (%)	G7 (%)	Paris Club (%)	Portland 30 (%)	Anglophone (%)
UK % of Population	0.0	0.1	0.1	0.1	0.1	0.1	0.1	0.1	0.1	0.1	0.1	0.1	0.0	0.1	0.1	0.0	0.1
Jan 1 2020 to June 30 2020	1.6	0.8	1.0	1.1	0.8	0.8	0.9	0.8	0.8	1.0	1.3	0.9	0.6	2.1	0.8	0.7	0.8
Jan 1 2020 to Dec 31 2020	2.6	1.2	1.7	1.3	1.1	1.1	1.3	1.1	1.1	2.0	2.0	1.3	0.9	4.0	1.3	1.0	1.2
Jan 1 2021 to Dec 31 2021	5.3	1.5	1.5	1.4	1.3	1.4	1.8	1.4	1.4	3.9	2.7	1.7	1.2	7.4	1.8	1.7	1.5
Jan 1 2022 to June 30 2022	17.5	4.8	7.0	3.3	4.7	4.8	5.6	4.7	4.6	13.0	9.6	4.5	4.3	17.0	5.5	5.4	4.3
Jan 1 2020 to June 30 2022	4.0	1.2	2.1	1.4	1.3	1.3	1.6	1.3	1.3	3.1	2.5	1.5	1.1	6.7	1.6	1.3	1.4

Source John Hopkins University Center for Systems Science and Engineering (CSSE) COVID-19 Data Repository and The Economist excess deaths tracker—https://www.economist.com/graphic-detail/coronavirus-excess-deaths-tracker

REFERENCES

Aglietta, M. (1979). *A theory of capitalist regulation.* New Left Books.

Arendt, H. (1958). *The human condition.* University of Chicago Press.

Arendt, H. (1963). *On revolution.* Viking Press.

Arendt, H. (1968). *Between past and future: Eight exercises in political thought.* Viking Press.

Arestis, P., & Sawyer, M. (2005). The neoliberal experience in the United Kingdom. In A. Saad-Filho & D. Johnston (Eds.), *Neoliberalism: A critical reader* (pp. 199–207). Pluto Press.

Audickas, L. et al. (2019). *Membership of UK political parties.*https://commonsli brary.parliament.uk/research-briefings/sn05125/. Accessed 18 August 2021.

Barry, J. (2021). Green republicanism and a 'Just Transition' from the tyranny of economic growth. *Critical Review of International Social and Political Philosophy, 24*(5), 725–742.

Bambra, C., Riordan, R., Ford, J., & Matthews, F. (2020). The COVID-19 pandemic and health inequalities. *Journal of Epidemiology and Community Health, 74*(11), 964–968.

BBC News. (2021). Covid inquiry: When will it happen and how does it work? https://www.bbc.co.uk/news/explainers-57085964. Accessed 28 Dec 2021.

Bell, T., & Brewer, M. (2021). *The 12-month stretch: Where the government has delivered—and where it has failed—during the Covid-19 crisis.* Resolution Foundation.

Bell, T., et al. (2021). *The Boris budget: Resolution Foundation analysis of autumn budget and spending review 2021.* Resolution Foundation.

Berlin, I. (1969). *Four essays on liberty.* Oxford University Press.

Berry, C. (2019). From receding to reseeding: Industrial policy, governance strategies and neoliberal resilience in post-crisis Britain. *New Political Economy, 25*(4), 607–625.

Beveridge, F. (2020). *Inequality in the Face of COVID-19: How do we Build Back Stronger in the Liverpool City Region?* University of Liverpool Heseltine Institute Policy Brief 27.

Boas, T. C., & Gans-Morse, J. (2009). Neoliberalism: From new liberal philosophy to anti-liberal slogan. *Studies in Comparative International Development, 44*, 137–161.

Brenner, N., & Theodore, N. (2002). Cities and the geographies of "Actually existing neoliberalism". *Antipode, 34*(3), 349–379.

Briggs, A., et al. (2020). NHS test and trace: The journey so far. https://www.health.org.uk/publications/long-reads/nhs-test-and-trace-the-journey-so-far. Accessed 28 Dec 2021.

Brown, W. (2005). *Edgework: Critical essays on knowledge and politics*. Princeton University Press.

Brown, W. (2015). *Undoing the demos: Neoliberalism's stealth revolution*. Zone Books.

Brown, J., & Kirk-Wade, E. (2021). *Coronavirus: A history of English lockdown laws* (Briefing Paper No. 9068). House of Commons Library.

Burnham, P. (2001). New Labour and the politics of depoliticization. *British Journal of Politics and International Relations, 3*(2), 127–149.

Buscha, F., Gorman, E., & Sturgis, P. (2021). Spatial and social mobility in England and Wales: A sub-national analysis of differences and trends over time. *British Journal of Sociology, 72*(5), 1378–1393.

Calvert, J., & Arbuthnott, G. (2021). *Failures of state: The inside story of Britain's battle with coronavirus*. HarperCollins.

Campbell, J. L., & Pedersen, O. K. (2001). *The rise of neoliberalism and institutional analysis*. Princeton University Press.

Christakis, N. A. (2020). *Apollo's arrow: The profound and enduring impact of coronavirus on the way we live*. Hachette London.

Clark, H. (2021). Examining the end of the furlough scheme. https://commonslibrary.parliament.uk/examining-the-end-of-the-furlough-scheme/. Accessed 28 Dec 2021.

Coffee, A. M. S. J. (2015). Two spheres of domination: Republican theory, social norms and the insufficiency of negative freedom. *Contemporary Political Theory, 14*(1), 45–62.

Collinson, P. (2017). Tax on test: Do Britons pay more than most? https://www.theguardian.com/money/2017/may/27/tax-britons-pay-europe-australia-us. Accessed 28 Dec 2021.

Committee on Climate Change (CCC). (2021). 2021 progress report to parliament. https://www.theccc.org.uk/publication/2021-progress-report-to-par liament/. Accessed 12 May 2022.

Costa, M. (2013). Is Neo-republicanism bad for women? *Hypatia, 28*(4), 921–936.

Cumbers, A. (2020). *The case for economic democracy.* Polity Press Bristol.

D'Ancona, M. (2020). Hancock is GREAT. https://members.tortoisemedia. com/2020/10/05/201005-test-and-trace-slow-news-audio-hancock-is-great-plus-transcript/content.html. Accessed 28 Dec 2021.

Dean, J. (2009). Democracy and other neoliberal fantasies. In *Democracy and other neoliberal fantasies.* Duke University Press.

Davies, M. (2002). *Late Victorian Holocausts: El Niño Famines and the Making of the Third World.* Verso.

Department for Business, Energy & Industrial Strategy. (2020). *Trade Union Membership, UK 1995-2019: Statistical Bulletin.*https://assets.publishing. service.gov.uk/government/uploads/system/uploads/attachment_data/file/ 887740/Trade-union-membership-2019-statistical-bulletin.pdf. Accessed 18 August 2021.

Dorey, P. (2015). A farewell to alms: Thatcherism's legacy of inequality. *British Politics, 10*(1), 79–98.

Eatwell, R. & Goodwin, M. (2018). *National populism: The revolt against liberal democracy.* Pelican.

Entwistle, V., Carter, S., & Little, M. (2016). Defending public health against 'nanny state' accusations: We need to talk about freedom. https://chpi. org.uk/blog/defending-public-health-nanny-state-accusations-need-talk-fre edom/ Accessed 2 May 2022.

Esping-Andersen, G. (1990). *The three worlds of welfare capitalism.* Princeton University Press.

European Centre for Disease Prevention and Control [ECDC]. (2021). *COVID-19 situation update worldwide, as of week 43,* updated 4 Nov 2021. https://www.ecdc.europa.eu/en/geographical-distribution-2019-ncov-cases. Accessed 28 Dec 2021.

Evans, J. (2021). From stay at home, stay alert and back to stay at home: How government's lockdown messaging changed over the last year. https://www. itv.com/news/2021-03-21/from-stay-at-home-stay-alert-and-back-to-stay-at-home-how-governments-lockdown-messaging-changed-over-the-last-year. Accessed 28 Dec 2021.

Exeter, D., Paynter, J., & Bullen, C. (2020). Going hard and going early in New Zealand: The "team of 5 million" unites against COVID-19. https://www. liverpool.ac.uk/media/livacuk/publicpolicyamppractice/covid-19/PB024. pdf. Accessed 28 Dec 2021.

Ferguson, N. (2021). *Doom: The politics of catastrophe.* Penguin.

Fisher, M. (2009). *Capitalist realism: Is there no alternative?* Zero Books.

Fisher-Pearson, N., & Mallet, J. (2020). Unmasking the Failings: Why the UK government was too slow on face coverings. https://cherwell.org/2020/08/09/unmasking-the-failings-why-the-uk-government-was-too-slow-on-face-coverings/. Accessed 28 Dec 2021.

Friedman, M. (1987). Free markets and free speech. *Harvard Journal of Law and Public Policy, 10*(1), 1–10.

Gallie, W. B. (1956). Essentially contested concepts. *Proceedings of the Aristotelian Society, 56,* 167–198.

Gallo, E. (2022). Three varieties of Authoritarian neoliberalism: Rule by the experts, the people, the leader. *Competition & Change, 26*(5), 554–574.

Galloway, L. (2020). Building a domestic manufacturing capacity. http://www.pharmatimes.com/web_exclusives/Building_a_domestic_manufacturing_capacity_1341929 Accessed 28 Dec 2021.

Geoghegan, P., et al. (2020). Revealed: 'Failing' Serco won another £57m COVID contract without competition. https://www.opendemocracy.net/en/dark-money-investigations/revealed-failing-serco-won-another-57m-covid-contract-without-competition/. Accessed 28 Dec 2021.

Giroux, H. A. (2021). The Covid-19 Pandemic is exposing the plague of neoliberalism. In N. K. Denzin and M. D. Giardina (Eds.), *Collaborative futures in qualitative inquiry research in a pandemic,* 17–26. Routledge.

Glover, R. E., & Maani, N. (2020). Have we reached "peak neoliberalism" in the UK's covid-19 response? https://blogs.bmj.com/bmj/2021/01/27/have-we-reached-peak-neoliberalism-in-the-uks-covid-19-response/. Accessed 28 Dec 2021.

Giddens, A. (1998). *The third way: The renewal of social democracy.* Polity

Giddens, A. (2000). *The third way and its critics.* Polity.

Gov.uk. (2021, May 12). PM house of commons statement on COVID. https://www.gov.uk/government/speeches/pm-house-of-commons-statement-on-covid-12-may-2021. Accessed 28 Dec 2021.

Gov.uk. (n.d.). Coronavirus (COVID-19) in the UK. https://coronavirus.data.gov.uk/. Accessed 28 Dec 2021.

Gourevitch, A. (2015). *From slavery to cooperative commonwealth: Labor and republican liberty in the nineteenth century.* Cambridge University Press.

Gray, M., & Barford, A. (2018). The depths of the cuts: The uneven geography of local government austerity. *Cambridge Journal of Regions, Economy and Society, 11*(3), 541–563.

Gurdasani, D., Drury, J., Greenhalgh, T., et al. (2021). Correspondence mass infection is not an option: We must do more to protect our young. *Lancet, 398*(10297), 297–298. https://doi.org/10.1016/S0140-6736(21)01589-0

Hacker, J. (2006). *The great risk shift: The new economic insecurity and the decline of the American dream.* Oxford University Press.

Hale, T., et al. (2020). *Variation in government responses to COVID-19* (BSG Working Paper Series, 2020/032), pp. 1–29.

Hall, S. (2011). The neoliberal revolution. *Soundings, 48*, 9–27.

Hall, P. A., & Soskice, D. (Eds.). (2001). *Varieties of capitalism: The institutional foundations of comparative advantage*. OUP.

Hanlon, P. (2015). Unhealthy glasgow: A case for ecological public health?. *Public Health, 129*(10), 1353–1360.

Hansard, H. C. (2021, June 30). Deb (vol. 698, col. 256).

Hansard, H. C. (2022, April 27). Deb (vol. 712, col. 755).

Harvey, D. (2003). *The new imperialism*. Oxford University Press.

Harvey, D. (2005). *A brief history of neoliberalism*. Oxford University Press.

Harvey, D. (2010). *The enigma of capital and the crises of capitalism*. Oxford University Press.

Harvey, D. (2007). Neoliberalism as creative destruction. *The ANNALS of the American Academy of Political and Social Science, 610*(1), 21–44.

Health and Social Care and Science and Technology Committees. (2021). *Coronavirus: Lessons learned to date* (HC 2021–22, 92). House of Commons.

Hecht, K., McArthur, D., Savage, M., & Friedman, S. (2020). *Elites in the UK: Pulling away?* The Sutton Trust.

HM Government. (2022). Covid-19 response: Living with Covid-19. https://assets.publishing.service.gov.uk/government/uploads/system/uploads/attachment_data/file/1056229/COVID-19_Response_-_Living_with_COVID-19.pdf. Accessed 12 May 2022.

HM Treasury. (2022). Government support for the cost of living: Factsheet. https://www.gov.uk/government/publications/government-support-for-the-cost-of-living-factsheet/government-support-for-the-cost-of-living-factsheet. Accessed 12 May 2022.

Hobbes, T. (2008). *Leviathan*. Oxford University Press.

Horton, R. (2020). *The COVID-19 catastrophe: What's gone wrong and how to stop it happening again*. Polity Press.

Horton, R., (2021). *The COVID-19 catastrophe: What's gone wrong and how to stop it happening again*. John Wiley & Sons.

Home Affairs Committee. (2020). *Home office preparedness for COVID-19 (coronavirus): Management of the borders* (HC 2019–21, 563). House of Commons.

Institute for Government [IfG]. (2021). Timeline of UK coronavirus lockdowns, March 2020 to March 2021. https://www.instituteforgovernment.org.uk/sites/default/files/timeline-lockdown-web.pdf. Accessed 28 Dec 2021.

Institute for Government. (2022). Cost of living crisis. https://www.instituteforgovernment.org.uk/explainers/cost-living-crisis. Accessed 12 May 2022.

Intergovernmental Panel on Climate Change [IPCC]. (2022). Climate Change 2022 mitigation of Climate Change: Summary for policymakers. https://report.ipcc.ch/ar6wg3/pdf/IPCC_AR6_WGIII_SummaryForPolicymakers.pdf. Accessed 12 May 2022.

Irving, S. (2020). Hayek's neo-Roman liberalism. *European Journal of Political Theory, 19*(4), 553–570.

James, T. (2018). Chapter 2.4: Are UK elections conducted with integrity, with sufficient turnout? In P. Dunleavy, et al. (Eds.), *The UK's Changing Democracy*. LSE Press, pp. 78–89.

Jefferies, S., et al. (2020). COVID-19 in New Zealand and the impact of the national response: A descriptive epidemiological study. *Lancet Public Health, 5*, e612–e623.

Johns, M. (2020). 10 years of austerity: Eroding resilience in the north. https://www.ippr.org/files/2020-06/10-years-of-austerity.pdf. Accessed 16 Dec 2021.

Johnson, B. (2020a, March 20). Prime Minister's statement on coronavirus (COVID-19). https://www.gov.uk/government/speeches/pm-statement-on-coronavirus-20-march-2020a. Accessed 28 Dec 2021.

Johnson, B. (2020b, September 22). PM Commons statement on coronavirus. https://www.gov.uk/government/speeches/pm-commons-statement-on-coronavirus-22-september-2020b. Accessed 28 Dec 2021.

Johnson, B. (2020c, December 16). Prime Minister's statement on coronavirus (COVID-19). https://www.gov.uk/government/speeches/prime-ministers-statement-on-coronavirus-covid-19-16-december-2020c. Accessed 28 Dec 2021.

Johnson, B. (2021a, February 22). PM statement to the House of Commons on roadmap for easing lockdown restrictions in England. https://www.gov.uk/government/speeches/pm-statement-to-the-house-of-commons-on-roadmap-for-easing-lockdown-restrictions-in-england-22-february-2021a. Accessed 28 Dec 2021.

Johnson, B. (2021b, July 19). PM statement at coronavirus press conference. https://www.gov.uk/government/speeches/pm-statement-at-coronavirus-press-conference-19-july-2021b. Accessed 28 Dec 2021.

Joseph Rowntree Foundation. (2020). *UK poverty 2019/20*. Joseph Rowntree Foundation.

Kettell, S., & Kerr, P. (2021). 'Guided by the science': (De)politicising the UK government's response to the coronavirus crisis. *The British Journal of Politics and International Relations, 24*(1), 11–30.

Kitchin, R. (2020). Civil liberties or public health, or civil liberties and public health? Using surveillance technologies to tackle the spread of COVID-19. *Space and Polity, 24*(3), 362–381.

Kitson, M., & Michie, J. (2014). *The deindustrial revolution: The rise and fall of UK manufacturing, 1870–2010* (Centre for Business Research, University of Cambridge Working Paper, 459), pp. 1–38.

Klein, N. (2020). *On fire: The (burning) case for a green new deal.* Simon & Schuster.

Laborde, C. (2008). *Critical republicanism: The Hijab controversy and political philosophy.* Oxford University Press.

Lee, P., et al. (2020). What we can learn from Taiwan's response to the covid-19 epidemic. https://blogs.bmj.com/bmj/2020/07/21/what-we-can-learn-from-taiwans-response-to-the-covid-19-epidemic/. Accessed 28 Dec 2021.

Lefkowitz, D. (2014). Strains of commitment. In J. Mandle & D. A. Reidy (Eds.), *The Cambridge Rawls Lexicon* (pp. 813–816). Cambridge University Press.

Leipold, B. (2020). Marx's social republic: Radical republicanism and the political institutions of socialism. In B. Leipold, K. Nabulsi, & S. White (Eds.), *Radical republicanism: Recovering the tradition's popular heritage* (pp. 172–193). Oxford University Press.

Leipold, B., Nabulsi, K., & White, S. (2020). *Radical republicanism: Recovering the tradition's popular heritage.* Oxford University Press.

Lovett, F. (2010). *A general theory of domination.* Oxford University Press.

Lovett, F., & Pettit, P. (2009). Neorepublicanism: A normative and institutional research program. *Annual Review of Political Science, 12*(1), 11–29.

Maconie, S. (2020). *The Nanny state made me.* Ebury Press.

MacGilvray, E. (2011). *The invention of market freedom.* Cambridge University Press.

Majeed, A., et al. (2020). Can the UK emulate the South Korean approach to covid-19? https://www.bmj.com/content/369/bmj.m2084. Accessed 28 Dec 2021.

Marmot, M. (2010). *Fair society, Healthy lives*: Strategic review of health inequalities in England post 2010. Marmot Review.

Marmot, M., et al. (2020). *Health equity in England: The Marmot review 10 years on.* Institute of Health Equity.

Martin, R., Gardiner, B., Pike, A., Sunley, P., & Tyler, P. (2021). *Levelling up left behind places: The scale and nature of the economic and policy challenge.* Routledge.

Mazzucato, M., & Kattel, R. (2020). COVID-19 and public-sector capacity. *Oxford Review of Economic Policy, 36*, S256–S269. https://doi.org/10.1093/oxrep/graa031

McCann, P. (2016). *The UK regional-national economic problem: Geography, globalisation and governance.* Routledge.

McCann, P. (2020). Perceptions of regional inequality and the geography of discontent: Insights from the UK. *Regional Studies, 54*(2), 256–267.

McCann, P. (2022). Raquel Ortega-Argilés, and Pei-Yu Yuan. "The Covid-19 shock in European regions." *Regional Studies, 56*(7), 1142–1160.

McCann, P., & Ortega-Argilés, R. (2021). The UK 'geography of discontent': Narratives, Brexit and inter-regional 'levelling up.' *Cambridge Journal of Regions, Economy and Society, 14*(3), 545–564.

McCormick, J. P. (2011). *Machiavellian democracy*. Cambridge University Press.

McGrane, D., & Hibbert, N. (2019). Introduction. In D. McGrane & N. Hibbert (Eds.), *Applied political theory and Canadian politics* (pp. 3–18). University of Toronto Press.

McKee, M. (2020). England's PPE procurement failures must never happen again. https://www.bmj.com/content/370/bmj.m2858. Accessed 28 Dec 2021.

Milanovic, B. (2019). Capitalism, alone: The future of the system that rules the world. Harvard University Press.

Mill, J. S. (2008). *On liberty and other essays*. Oxford University Press.

Mellish, T. I., Luzmore, N. J., & Shahbaz, A. A. (2020). Why were the UK and USA unprepared for the COVID-19 pandemic? The systemic weaknesses of neoliberalism: A comparison between the UK, USA, Germany, and South Korea. *Journal of Global Faultlines, 7*(1), 9–45.

Ministry of Health and Welfare. (2020). COVID-19 response. http://ncov.mohw.go.kr/en/baroView.do?brdId=11&brdGubun=111&dataGubun=&ncvContSeq=&contSeq=&board_id=. Accessed 28 Dec 2021.

Mouffe, C. (2000). *The democratic paradox*. Verso.

Mouffe, C. (2005). *On the political*.Routledge.

Mouffe, C. (2013). *Agonistics*. Verso.

Munck, R. (2005). Neoliberalism and politics, and the politics of neoliberalism. In A. Saad-Filho & D. Johnston (Eds.), *Neoliberalism: A critical reader* (pp. 60–69). Pluto Press.

Mudge, S. L. (2008). What is neo-liberalism? *Socio-Economic Review, 6*, 703–731.

Näsström, S., & Kalm, S. (2015). A democratic critique of precarity. *Global Discourse, 5*(4), 556–573.

National Audit Office [NAO]. (2013). The role of major contractors in the delivery of public services. https://www.nao.org.uk/wp-content/uploads/2013/11/10296-001-Delivery-of-public-services-HC-8101.pdf. Accessed 28 Dec 2021.

National Audit Office [NAO]. (2016). *Benefit sanctions*. National Audit Office.

Navarro, V. (2020). The consequences of neoliberalism in the current pandemic. *International Journal of Health Services, 50*(3), 271–275.

Nelson, E. (2020). Britain's new record: A Recession worse than in Europe and North America. https://www.nytimes.com/2020/08/12/business/britain-economy-recession-coronavirus.html?auth=login-email&login=email. Accessed 28 Dec 2021.

Nice, A. (2020). Extraordinary coronavirus restrictions on personal freedom require proper parliamentary scrutiny. https://www.instituteforgovernment.org.uk/blog/coronavirus-restrictions-parliamentary-scrutiny. Accessed 28 Dec 2021.

Nozick, R. (1974). *Anarchy, state, and utopia*. Blackwell.

Office for Budget Responsibility [OBR]. (2021). *Economic and fiscal outlook, October 2021* (CP 545). Her Majesty's Stationery Office.

O'Shea, T. (2020). In defence of public ownership: A reply to Frye. *Political Theory, 48*(5), 581–587.

Painter, A. (2020). Coronavirus: Respond at scale, build bridges to the future. https://www.thersa.org/blog/2020/03/coronavirus-respond-at-scale-build-bridges-to-the-future. Accessed 12 May 2022.

Pettit, P. (1996). Freedom as anti-power. *Ethics, 106*(3), 576–604.

Pettit, P. (1997). *Republicanism: A theory of freedom and government*. Oxford University Press.

Pettit, P. (2002). Keeping republican freedom simple: On a difference with Quentin Skinner. *Political Theory, 30*(3), 339–356.

Pettit, P. (2007). A republican right to basic income? *Basic Income Studies, 2*(2), 1–8.

Pettit, P. (2010). Civic republican theory. In J. L. Martí & P. Pettit (Eds.), *A political philosophy in public life: Civic republicanism in Zapatero's Spain*. Princeton University Press.

Pettit, P. (2012). *On the people's terms: A republican theory and model of democracy*. Cambridge University Press.

Peck, J. (2010). *Constructions of neoliberal reason*. OUP.

Peck, J. (2013). Explaining (with) neoliberalism. *Territory, Politics, Governance, 1*(2), 132–157.

Peck, J. (2022). Confessions of a recovering régulation theorist. In B. Hillier, R. Philips & J. Peck (Eds.), *Regulation theory, space, and uneven development* (pp. 169–190). 1984Press.

Peck, J., & Theodore, N. (2019). Still neoliberalism? *South Atlantic Quarterly, 118*(2), 245–265.

Peck, J., Theodore, N., & Brenner, N. (2013). Neoliberal urbanism redux? *International Journal of Urban and Regional Research, 37*(3), 1091–1099.

Piketty, T. (2020). *Capital and ideology*. Harvard University Press.

Phelan, S. (2022). What's in a name? Political antagonism and critiquing 'neoliberalism'. *Journal of Political Ideologies, 27*(2), 148–167.

Piketty, T. (2014). *Capital in the twenty-first century, Thomas Piketty*. Cambridge, MA.

Piketty, T. (2020). *Capital and ideology*. Cambridge, MA.

Piketty, T. (2022). A brief history of equality. Harvard University Press.

Piore, M., & Sabel, C. F. (1984). *The second industrial divide: Possibilities for prosperity*. Basic Books.

Pocock, J. G. A. (2003). *The machiavellian moment*. Princeton University Press.

Ranciere, J. (1995). *On the shores of politics*. Verso.

Ranciere, J. (1999). *Disagreement: Politics and philosophy*. University of Minnesota Press.

Rancière, J. (2004). *The politics of aesthetics: The distribution of the sensible*. Continuum London.

Ranciere, J. (2006). *Hatred of democracy*. Verso.

Rawlinson, K. (2020). Coronavirus PPE: All 400,000 gowns flown from Turkey for NHS fail UK standards. https://www.theguardian.com/world/2020/may/07/all-400000-gowns-flown-from-turkey-for-nhs-fail-uk-standards. Accessed 28 Dec 2021.

Rawls, J. (2001). *Justice as fairness: A restatement*. Harvard University Press.

Raworth, K. (2017). *Doughnut economics: Seven ways to think like a 21st-century economist*. Chelsea Green Publishing.

Resolution Foundation. (2022). Inflation nation: Putting spring statement 2022 in context. https://www.resolutionfoundation.org/publications/inflation-nation/. Accessed 12 May 2022.

Rhodes, C., Hough, D., & Butcher, L. (2014). *Privatisation* (Research Paper No. 14/61). House of Commons Library.

Roy, A. (2020). The pandemic is a portal. https://www.ft.com/content/10d8f5e8-74eb-11ea-95fe-fcd274e920ca. Accessed 12 May 2022.

Saad-Filho, A. (2020). From COVID-19 to the end of neoliberalism. *Critical Sociology, 46*, 477–485.

Saad-Filho, A. (2021). Endgame: From crisis in neoliberalism to crises of neoliberalism. *Human Geography, 14*(1), 133–137.

Salerno, M., Hyseni, L., Bickerstaffe, H., Capwell, S., & Lloyd-Williams, F. (2020). OP61 Media analysis of the term 'Nanny State' in UK print and online newspapers: Implications for public health advocacy. *Journal of Epidemiology & Community Health, 74*(1), A29.

Sample, I., & Stewart, H. (2021). Bring in measures soon or risk 7,000 daily Covid hospitalisations. *Sage warns*. https://www.theguardian.com/world/2021/sep/14/bring-in-measures-soon-or-risk-7000-daily-covid-cases-sage-warns. Accessed 28 Dec 2021.

Scally, G., Jacobsen, B., & Abbasi, K. (2020). The UK's public health response to covid-19. https://www.bmj.com/content/369/bmj.m1932. Accessed 28 Dec 2021.

Schofield, J., Leelarathna, L. & Thabit, H. (2020). COVID- 19: Impact of and on diabetes. *Diabetes Therapy, 11*(7), 1429–1435.

Sen, A. (1999). *Development as freedom*. Knopf.

Singer, M. (2009). *Introduction to syndemics: A critical systems approach to public and community health*. John Wiley & Sons.

Skinner, Q. (2012). *Liberty before liberalism*. Cambridge University Press.

Smith, N. (1984). Uneven development: Nature, capital, and the production of space. Blackwell.

Smith, N. (2006). There's no such thing as a natural disaster. https://items.ssrc.org/understanding-katrina/theres-no-such-thing-as-a-natural-disaster/. Accessed 28 Dec 2021.

Smits, K. (2016). *Applying political theory*. Palgrave.

Sparke, M., & Williams, O. D. (2022). Neoliberal disease: COVID-19, co-pathogenesis and global health insecurities. *Environment and Planning A: Economy and Space, 54*(1), 15–32.

Springer, S. (2010). Neoliberalism and geography: Expansions, variegations, formations. *Geography Compass, 4*(8), 1025–1038.

Springer, S. (2016). Fuck neoliberalism. *ACME: An International Journal for Critical Geographies, 15*(2), 285–292.

Springer, S. (2021). *Fuck neoliberalism: Translating resistance*. PM Press.

Standing, G. (2011). *The precariat: The new dangerous class*. Bloomsbury.

Standring, A., & Davies, J. (2020). From crisis to catastrophe: The death and viral legacies of austere neoliberalism in Europe? *Dialogues in Human Geography, 10*(2), 146–149.

Sultana, F. (2021). Climate change, COVID-19, and the co-production of injustices: A feminist reading of overlapping crises. *Social & Cultural Geography, 22*(4), 447–460.

Šumonja, M. (2021). Neoliberalism is not dead–On political implications of Covid-19. *Capital & Class, 45*(2), 215–227.

Swyngedouw, E. (2009). The antinomies of the postpolitical city: In search of a democratic politics of environmental production. *International Journal of Urban and Regional Research, 33*(3), 601e620.

Tatlow, H. et al. (2021). Variation in the response to COVID-19 across the four nations of the United Kingdom. https://www.bsg.ox.ac.uk/sites/default/files/2021-04/BSG-WP-2020-035-v2.0.pdf. Accessed 28 Dec 2021.

Taylor, F.W. (1911). *The principles of scientific management*. Harper & Brothers.

Taylor, R. S. (2017). *Exit left: Markets and mobility in republican thought*. Oxford University Press.

Thatcher, M. (1968). Conservative political centre (CPC) lecture ("what's wrong with politics?"). https://www.margaretthatcher.org/document/101632. Accessed 28 Dec 2021.

The King's Fund. (2020). Public health: Our position. https://www.kingsfund. org.uk/projects/positions/public-health. Accessed 28 Dec 2021.

The Organisation for Economic Co-operation and Development [OECD]. (2020). *Policy responses to coronavirus (COVID-19) the territorial impact of COVID-19: Managing the crisis across levels of government.* OECD.

The Organisation for Economic Co-operation and Development [OECD]. (2021). *Government at a glance.* OECD.

The Scottish Parliament. (2021). Citizens' panel convened to discuss Scotland Covid-19 restrictions and strategy. https://archive2021.parliament.scot/new sandmediacentre/116952.aspx. Accessed 28 Dec 2021.

The Treasury. (2019). The wellbeing budget 2019. https://www.treasury.govt. nz/publications/wellbeing-budget/wellbeing-budget-2019-html.   Accessed 13 May 2022.

The Treasury. (2021). Wellbeing budget 2021: Securing our recovery. https:// www.treasury.govt.nz/publications/wellbeing-budget/wellbeing-budget-2021-securing-our-recovery. Accessed 13 May 2022.

Theodore, N., Peck, J., & Brenner, N. (2011). Neoliberal urbanism: Cities and the rule of markets. In G. Bridge & S. Watson (Eds.), *The New Blackwell companion to the city* (pp. 15–25). Wiley Blackwell.

Thomas, C. (2019). *Hitting the poorest worst? How public health cuts have been experienced in England's most deprived communities.* https://www.ippr.org/ blog/public-health-cuts. Accessed 9 Nov 2022.

Thorsen, D. E. (2010). The neoliberal challenge: What is neoliberalism? *Contemporary Readings in Law and Social Justice, 2*(2), 188–214.

Tomasi, J. (2012). *Free market fairness.* Princeton University Press.

Trades Union Congress [TUC]. (2021). Sick pay that works. https://www.tuc. org.uk/research-analysis/reports/sick-pay-works Accessed 28 Dec 2021.

UK2070. (2020). *Make no little plans: Acting at scale for a fairer and stronger future.* UK2070 Commission.

United Nations [UN]. (2019). Visit to the United Kingdom of Great Britain and Northern Ireland: Report of the special rapporteur on extreme poverty and human rights. https://undocs.org/A/HRC/41/39/Add.1. Accessed 28 Dec 2020.

Vallier, K. (2021). Neoliberalism. https://plato.stanford.edu/archives/sum 2021/entries/neoliberalism/. Accessed 28 Dec 2021.

Venugopal, R. (2015). Neoliberalism as concept. *Economy and Society, 44*(2), 165–187.

Vize, R. (2020) How the erosion of our public health system hobbled England's covid-19 response. https://www.bmj.com/content/369/bmj. m1934. Accessed 28 Dec 2021.

Wang, B., Li, R., Lu, Z. & Huang, Y. (2020). *Does comorbidity increase the risk of patients with COVID-19: Evidence from meta-analysis, 12*(7), 6049. Aging (Albany NY).

Wilkinson, R., & Pickett, K. (2010). *The spirit level: Why equality is better for everyone.* Penguin.

Wilkinson, R., & Pickett, K. (2020). *The inner level: How more equal societies reduce stress, restore sanity and improve everyone's well-being.* Penguin.

Williams, G. A., Rajan, R., & Cylus, J. D. (2021). Covid-19 in the United Kingdom: How austerity and a loss of state capacity undermined the crisis response. In S. L. Greer, E. J. King, E. M. da Fonseca, & A. Peralta-Santos (Eds.), *Coronavirus politics: The comparative politics and policy of COVID-19* (pp. 215–234). University of Michigan Press.

World Health Organisation [WHO]. (2020a, March 5). WHO Director-General's opening remarks at the media briefing on COVID-19. https:// www.who.int/director-general/speeches/detail/who-director-general-s-ope ning-remarks-at-the-media-briefing-on-covid-19---5-march-2020a. Accessed 5 May 2022.

World Health Organisation [WHO]. (2020b, March 16). WHO Director-General's opening remarks at the media briefing on COVID-19. https:// www.who.int/dg/speeches/detail/who-director-general-s-opening-remarks-at-the-media-briefing-on-covid-19---16-march-2020b. Accessed   28   Dec 2021.

Wright, S., Fletcher, D. R., & Stewart, A. B. R. (2020). Punitive benefit sanctions, welfare conditionality, and the social abuse of unemployed people in Britain: Transforming claimants into offenders? *Social Policy & Administration, 54*(2), 278–294.

Žižek, S. (1999). *The Ticklish subject: The absent centre of political ontology.* Verso.

DATA SETS

Economist coronavirus-excess-deaths-tracker. https://www.economist.com/gra phic-detail/coronavirus-excess-deaths-tracker

European Centre for Disease Control and Prevention (ECDC). https://www. ecdc.europa.eu/en/coronavirus

European Union. https://www.europa.eu/european-union/coronavirus-respon se_en

Important websites providing authoritative data and analysis of COVID-19 and its geographies include:

International Monetary Fund. https://www.imf.org/en/Topics/imf-and-cov id19

Institute of Health Metrics and Evaluation. https://www.ghdx.healthdata.org/ record/ihme-data/covid_19_excess_mortality

Johns Hopkins University. https://www.coronavirus.jhu.edu/
Our World in Data. https://www.ourworldindata.org/coronavirus
The British Medical Journal. https://www.bmj.com/coronavirus
The Lancet Journal. https://www.thelancet.com/coronavirus
The Oxford COVID-19 Government Response Tracker (OxCGRT). https://www.covidtracker.bsg.ox.ac.uk/
The UK Office for National Statistics (ONS—in Scotland SNR and Northern Ireland NISRA). https://www.ons.org/coronavirus
Whitehead, M., McInroy, N., & Bambra, C. et al. (2014). *Due North report of the inquiry on health equity in the North*. Liverpool: University of Liverpool and the Centre for Economic Strategies.
Whitehead, M., Taylor-Robinson, D., & Barr, B. (2014). Great leap backwards. *British Medical Journal*, 349. https://doi.org/10.1136/bmj.g7350
World Bank. https://www.worldbank.org/en/topic/health/coronavirus
World Health Organization. https://www.who.int/
World Inequalities Database. https://www.wid.world/
US Centre for Disease Control and Prevention (CDC). https://www.cdc.gov/coronavirus/2019-nCoV/index.html

INDEX